CREATING WINNING GRANT PROPOSALS

Creating Winning Grant Proposals

A Step-by-Step Guide

Anne L. Rothstein

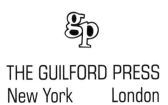

THE GUILFORD PRESS
New York   London

Copyright © 2019 The Guilford Press
A Division of Guilford Publications, Inc.
370 Seventh Avenue, Suite 1200, New York, NY 10001
www.guilford.com

Printed in the United States of America

This book is printed on acid-free paper.

Last digit is print number: 9   8   7   6   5   4   3   2   1

Library of Congress Cataloging-in-Publication Data is available from the publisher.

ISBN 978-1-4625-3908-6 (paperback)
ISBN 978-1-4625-3909-3 (hardcover)

This book is dedicated to the past, current, and future students and teachers whom proposals are intended to serve, and to those who are committed to devoting their time, effort, and expertise to writing them.

Most especially, I lovingly dedicate this book to Jane Hellman, who has supported and encouraged my lifelong passion for program development, proposal writing, and project oversight—despite the fact that they have often monopolized my time.

Preface

The process approach to proposal writing focuses on a set of systematic, organized, and thoughtful methods to conceptualize, design, write, edit, and finalize a competitive set of documents to submit to a funder. Accordingly, this book leads the reader/user systematically through the successive steps needed to prepare to write a proposal and then proceeds section by section to detail the steps needed to produce a complete competitive proposal. It is intended for use in proposal-writing workshops, in graduate courses that include topics in proposal writing, in proposal-writing courses, by individuals seeking to learn how to craft successful proposals, by more experienced proposal writers who want to improve, and by organizations that need to obtain funding for programmatic purposes. With practice, the steps to create a competitive proposal can become second nature.

The book is organized into three parts: Preparing for the Proposal, Elements of the Proposal, and Additional Considerations. In addition, there are practice exercises; 14 reproducible forms; a glossary of key terms; and five appendices, including one on action verbs, which are important in engaging the reader; web resources, organized by book chapter; examples of selection criteria; a sample memorandum of understanding; and tips for successful proposal writing. Each chapter begins with a list of learning objectives and ends with a summary section.

Part I. Preparing for the Proposal

Chapters 1–5 take the reader through the process of developing proposal topics based on the needs of the school, organization, or institution. Chapter 1 helps the reader determine whether his or her idea, the target population, research-based activities, organizational strengths, and the location of the project meet the requirements of the funding agency. The chapter also offers seven reasons why institutions and organizations should seek external funding. Chapter 2 highlights the tasks that are central to the exploration and development of potential projects that will serve your institution/organization. Emphasis is placed on the notion of "marketing" your idea to the funder. How does your idea contribute to the mission, vision, or purposes of the funder? Assuming that you have a project idea, how do you go about finding funding that will support your goals and objectives? In addition, several procedures for engaging groups of individuals and synthesizing their input are presented with examples of the process. This chapter also highlights the critical importance of establishing/proving need. Finally, the process of linking projects and matching projects to funding sources is presented. Highlighting the current emphasis on collaboration, Chapter 3 addresses some critical considerations in partnering with other institutions and organizations. In developing your specific proposal focus, Chapter 4 recommends that you consider all of the aspects of the project you are considering by first expanding/broadening your conception of what you will want to accomplish, how you will accomplish it, and how you will know that you have succeeded. Once you have a broad view you can begin to focus on the aspects that are realistically achievable, most critical to institutional success, appealing to funders, capacity building, and attainable. It is suggested that in some cases it is possible to submit multiple proposals to a funder if different populations are being served, and to submit the same project to different funders for different aspects of a program approach. An example focuses on increasing college readiness, access, and completion for first-generation low-income students. Finally, now that you have an idea for a proposal, you need to find a funding source. So Chapter 5 highlights several approaches to searching for Requests for Proposals (RFPs) and includes instructions for how to use Internet sites that provide funding information. There are 17 government funding agencies and 16 foundations presented, including website, overview, ways to find funding, eligibility, types of funding, application process, and other information.

Part II. Elements of the Proposal

The second section of the book is a systematic approach to the writing of the proposal and begins, in Chapter 6, with the creation of a Master Table that does not actually appear in the submitted proposal but is recommended to ensure that all tables presented throughout the proposal are consistent. The elements of the Master Table are Need, Objective, Activities, Description of Activity, Output, Outcomes, Evaluative Measures, and Responsible Individual. The Master Table is parsed into the various tables needed for other sections of the proposal. Chapter 7 provides an annotated summary of the proposal elements. This is followed by Chapter 8, which addresses the abstract and introduction and provides the reader with an overview of the project as well as the first view of the applicant. This enables the applicant to establish institutional/organizational credibility in relation to the proposal to be presented. Also in the introduction you are, for the first time, selling or positioning your institution as the best possible choice for achieving the goals and objectives proposed. Many RFPs require a logic model as part of the proposal narrative. Thus, Chapter 9 provides an overview and examples of logic models which demonstrate how the available resources contribute to the achievement of objectives through specific activities and how the activities lead to the short, mid- and long-term outcomes.

The first and most critical section of the proposal establishes the need for the project. This section is worth 24 out of 100 total points and has several specific items that must be included in a complete response. Chapter 10 describes several resources available on the Internet, including the U.S. Census American FactFinder site, that show how local data can be accessed and used in charts and tables to demonstrate high need. The examples include the types of explanations that are required so that the reader can interpret the data correctly. The data in this chapter lead directly to the goals and objectives section, covered in Chapter 11. For some RFPs, the objectives are provided within the selection criteria and all proposals must use the same objectives. However, the institution/organization has to consider the needs, available information about the population to be served, and the desired outcomes in order to establish reasonable percentages for the objectives. The TRIO proposal used as an example shows why the objective is ambitious and attainable: ambitious because of the need that is demonstrated, and attainable because of the activities and interventions to be implemented. Frequently, proposers will want to include a table that shows the need, objectives arising from those needs, activities to address the need and accomplish the objectives, and evaluative measures that will show how you know the objectives have been achieved.

The most valuable section of a proposal is the Plan of Operation (Chapter 12), worth 30 out of 100 points. It presents, in as much detail as page limits will allow, a road map to the implementation of the project. Each of the required subsections is illustrated and specifies the information required for the reader to ascertain the score to assign. I like to think of this section as a *cookbook for conducting the project*. This section of your proposal is usually the longest and most detailed. The reader must see the connections among this section, the need, goals, and objectives, and the budget. Parts of the Master Table will be appropriately used in this section. One of the most critical sections, the evaluation (covered in Chapter 13), is frequently left for last probably because it is at the end and worth only 5 points. Nevertheless, knowing how you will assess the outcomes of the project and thus determine whether your approach to resolving the need and realizing the objectives through the plan you will implement is central to achieving your goals. The goals, objectives, and evaluation measures presented in the Master Table should match those presented here. This chapter, by design, covers topics important to your understanding of evaluation and should be read thoroughly before starting on your section.

Once you have finished the sections that indicate what you will do to address the needs, achieve your objectives, and evaluate your success it is time to finalize the budget. At some point, when developing the Plan of Operation, you thought about who would conduct the project and what resources you might need for the activities you conduct and maybe even developed a preliminary budget. Chapter 14 takes you through the budget process and also considers the budget narrative. As with the evaluation section, the budget section is usually worth 5 or so points, but a few points often make the difference between proposals that meet the cutoff score and those that do not. The RFP always has a section on what expenses are allowed and what expenses are disallowed. This chapter provides needed details for shaping a meaningful budget narrative.

Part III. Additional Considerations

The third section of the book covers topics that, increasingly, are required by RFPs. These include sections on dissemination, sustainability, and significance (Chapter 15) and research-supported responses to invitational and competitive priorities (Chapter 16). So Chapter 15 provides information on how to disseminate your findings, and on steps you can take to sustain your work after funding ends and show that your project makes a significant contribution to knowledge in your field. Chapter 16 reveals the approved list of U.S. Department of Education priorities and explains where and how to find research studies illustrating that the activities and interventions you propose are supported by at least moderate evidence. Invitational priorities *must* be addressed to qualify for the competition but are not associated with point values. Competitive priorities, on the other hand, are assigned points based on the quality of the research you cite and how you relate the research to the activities you plan to implement. Although responding to competitive priorities is optional, failure to do so will severely impact your funding chances. Closing Part III, Chapter 17 provides in-depth information about the proposal review process. The best way to understand the review process is to sign up to be a peer reviewer. The USDE encourages individuals to submit their profile and provides a site where you can apply to read proposals. The site provided is for TRIO (*www2.ed.gov/about/offices/list/ope/trio/seekingfieldreaders.html*). You can also become familiar with the peer review process by studying the forms used to score proposals. You will see that they follow the selection criteria exactly and include the score values as well as fields for the reviewer to indicate proposal strengths and weaknesses. Chapter 17 presents a simulated review form as well as an actual review.

Chapter 18, the final chapter of the book, asks the question "What next?" This is intended to start you on your way by suggesting a series of steps you can take and contacts you can make to facilitate your proposal work. Here I also revisit the topic of why you should consider writing a proposal, in the hopes that you will use the information and examples provided in this book to start or to continue preparing successful proposals.

I have written this book to share my more than 35 years of experience learning to write proposals. Initially, in the 1980s and early 1990s, I wrote proposals to apply for state funding for what were, at the time, innovative and forward-looking programs. As I developed my insight and skill, I began to attend proposal-writing workshops to learn as much as I could about crafting winning proposals. Every workshop taught me something; I never stopped learning. Soon I was asked to speak at workshops to share my skills, knowledge, and insight. This "teaching" helped me learn even more; I had to organize the information, and the good questions of those attending made me think more about my process. I have been successful in receiving funding for my college because our borough (the Bronx, New York) has great needs that our proposals were able to articulate; we had ideas for innovative approaches to resolve these needs; objectives were based on need and were ambitious but attainable; our plan for implementation was solid; the evaluation was appropriate to the project; and the proposal was consistent. Still, a great proposal is not always selected for funding. So I continued to learn and to submit with the help of colleagues. I would estimate that over the past 35 years, I have submitted or collaborated on more than 400 proposals, of which more than 300 were funded. The college and my collaborators have received more than $300 million in funding, and many individuals have benefited.

Acknowledgments

For the past 35 years, I have collaborated with, sought advice from, and depended on many colleagues and friends who have helped conceptualize, create, write, edit, revise, and prepare more than 300 proposals that have received funding. The proposal examples presented in this book are the result of their many hours of work, discussion, review, and editing. I cannot thank them enough for allowing me to share their work with you. They have informed and assisted me in honing my writing skills in general and my proposal-writing skills in particular, encouraged me to think deeply about how best to serve local communities, and led me to make a commitment to the students who have benefited from engagement with school/college collaborative and college-based programs.

In 1984, when I was Associate Dean of Professional Studies at Lehman College, my Dean, Dr. Thomas K. Minter, urged me to complete a proposal, due in a week, which had been left unfinished by a faculty member. I did it, we were funded, and our project liaison, Michael Stevens, became a good friend and mentor who worked with me over the next 5 years to provide extensive, critical feedback on how to improve my proposals. He taught me many important lessons and strategies to ensure that readers could see how the parts of my proposals fit together and why our interventions would lead to positive outcomes for participants. My proposal-writing skills, particularly in the case of responding to TRIO RFPs, have benefited greatly from my participation in almost every proposal-writing workshop—staffed by outstanding speakers, especially Maureen Hoyler, Julia Tower, and Andrea Reeve—offered by the Council for Opportunity in Education, with the assistance of Angelica Vialpando, Vice President, Program and Professional Development; Nicole Norfles, Director, Program Practice and Innovation; and Neda Wickson, Program Assistant.

I also owe thanks to participating students who graciously responded to yearly surveys about their project experiences, and to instructors from the schools we served who gave up their summers and Saturdays to learn how to deliver project-based instruction and engage students to improve academic outcomes, increase student interest in science and math, and improve their college readiness and college access. Instructors also offered important feedback about how to better engage students, improve outcomes, and increase student retention and persistence.

Without the always supportive Lehman Office of Research and Sponsored Programs and the assistance of the late Barbara Bralver and the current director, Saeedah Hickman, as well as the knowledgeable support of Valerie Luria and Donnaree Smith, proposal submission might not have happened on time, on budget, and in required format. Their attention to detail, understanding of the RFP requirements, close attention to the budget and budget narrative, constant verification of budget accuracy, and expert transfer of all information for submission to funding agencies were central to timely mailing (in the past) and uploading (now).

I am grateful to the three presidents of Lehman College: the late Dr. Leonard Lief, Dr. Ricardo Fernandez, and our newest, Dr. Jose Luis Cruz, who believed that my proposal-writing skills were an asset to the college and provided the time and support for me to do what I do best. During the 1980s, when the City University of New York was experiencing budget problems, Dr. Lief asked me what I was going to do about it. I answered, "Write a proposal." I did, and Lehman was awarded a 5-year grant for over $2.1 million.

I also want to recognize the Deans of Education who supported and assisted me: Dr. Thomas K. Minter, mentioned previously, who got me started; Dr. James Bruni, who continuously encouraged and supported my work; Dr. Annette Digby, who had good advice and ideas; Dr. Susan Polirstok, who provided excellent ideas and suggestions; Dr. Deborah Eldridge, who shared her proposal-writing skills with me; Dr. Gaoyin Quin, Associate Dean; and Dr. Deborah Shanley, our most recent Dean, a friend for many years, who always had great ideas about activities and interventions that could be incorporated into proposals.

I owe a special heartfelt thank you to Dr. Harriet Fayne, Professor, Department of Counseling, Leadership, Literacy and Special Education, for her help and support in too many areas to be counted. Her understanding of program planning, proposal writing, and grant implementation and her willingness to read and edit have greatly improved the proposals submitted as well as, I believe, influenced the number of grant awards received.

I have also been fortunate to work with outstanding evaluators over the past several years who have contributed to my knowledge about research design and evaluation. These are Deb Coffey, Rebecca Eddy, and Monique Matelski.

My sincere appreciation goes to my friends and colleagues at Lehman who, over the years, have invited me to work on proposals with them; taught me so much about how to engage readers; invested their time and insight to share student stories, needs, and experiences; put forth the effort to conceptualize, design, and write parts of proposals; read, commented on, revised, and improved drafts; and worked to implement funded programs. These include Anne Johnson, retired as Vice President for Institutional Advancement; Eileen Allman, retired as Associate Professor of English; Paul Kreutzer, retired; Reine Sarmiento, Vice President for Enrollment Management; Jose Magdaleno, Vice President for Student Affairs; and Althea Forde, Ronald Banks, Richard Finger, Lisa Moalem, Laurie Austin, and Nancy Cintron. Without Susanne Tumelty, retired Vice President, and Michael Goldberg, Associate Director for Institutional Research, the extensive data required to support our needs would not have been available in timely fashion so often for so many proposals.

Current and former members of the Early Childhood and Childhood Education Department have contributed ideas, curriculum maps, activities, and research articles and written sections for the many proposals written to support work with preservice teachers and clinical residents. The proposals probably would not have been funded without the expertise of Abigail McNamee, Nancy Dubetz, Alexandria Ross, Cecilia Espinosa, Jennifer Collett, Anne Marie Marshall, and Andrea Zakin. Several individuals in other School of Education departments have been helpful by sharing ideas, research, concepts, and narratives. They are Wesley Pitts, Gillian Bayne, Serigne Gningue, and Joye Smith.

My fondest appreciation, however, is for the individuals who have worked in the Lehman Center for School/College Collaboratives over the past 35 years, supporting me, helping to prepare proposals, and doing the extensive and detailed work needed to manage funded projects. Thank you to Pedro Baez, Dena Rosario, Roz Krakowsky, Grace Colon, Traci Palmieri, Magali Figueroa-Sanchez, Phyllis McCabe, Phyllis Opochinsky, Laura Tringali, Kayla Castillo, Johanny Santiago, Thamar Pacheco, Desiree Barnes, and Dorothy Jacob. They have made it easy for me to focus on proposal writing and assisted in preparing charts and tables, structuring budgets, filling out proposal forms, checking formats and page numbers, creating tables of contents, and making sure that deadlines were met. Before grants.gov there were late-night runs to the local Federal Express office, to the Bronx Central Post Office, and once to the Manhattan Central Post Office right before midnight on the required mailing date.

Special gratitude and indebtedness go to C. Deborah Laughton and Katherine Sommer at The Guilford Press for their patience and assistance in shepherding this book to completion. My attention to deadlines is rather lax, unless it is for a proposal, which I always get out on time, so they were quite challenged. Those who reviewed the initial submitted manuscript—Susan Johnson, Community Resource and Development, Arizona State University; Vicki Jozefowicz, Public Administration, Eastern Kentucky University; David

Lotempio, Management, SUNY Buffalo; Binneh Minteh, Public Administration, Rutgers University; and Linda Silka, Policy Center, University of Maine—made it easy for me to follow their excellent suggestions and questions. I believe their input has greatly improved the expanded manuscript; their recommended changes have made the book more user-friendly, comprehensive, and better organized.

Despite all of the support and assistance I have received, the proposal-writing workshops I have attended, and all the rewrites and edits that have been suggested, this book is my responsibility, and I am accountable for its contents. My fondest wish is for readers to be assisted in writing more and better proposals that will serve the individuals in the United States who are most vulnerable and who need our support to grow, learn, and thrive.

We see what can be, believe that it can be done, and know that we have the power to do it.

Contents

PART III. Additional Considerations

PART I

Preparing for the Proposal

The Process Approach

HOW AND WHY

Individuals frequently use the term *grant writing* without realizing that a grant is the funding instrument issued by the agency, corporation, or foundation providing the money for the program. Individuals, colleges, and organizations submit a proposal to solicit funding for a project or program they have developed. Throughout this book, therefore, I will use the term *proposal* to refer to the document you prepare and submit.

Successful proposal writing can begin in a number of ways but always follows a **systematic process.** As will be seen in the chapter on developing the idea, a grant proposal can develop from *review of needs of the institution or population to be served*. It can also begin with *information about a successful program targeting a similar college* or group. You might also review published Requests for Proposals (RFPs) or recently awarded grants and find one that fits your students. Regardless of how you identify the source of funds and whether it is a federal, state, local, or a corporate source or a foundation, the

> **Proposal Ideas Can Develop from Different Approaches**
>
> Proposal ideas can develop from studying institutional needs, successful programs, Requests for Proposals, and/or recently awarded grants.

What Is an RFP?

An RFP is a document issued by a government agency, a corporate entity, or a charitable foundation inviting applications for funding. The RFP provides the rules, regulations, and framework to be followed in preparing a proposal.

What Is Scaffolding?

Scaffolding uses instructional techniques designed to build student knowledge, skills, and understanding through small steps that build upon one another.

A Grant Is Never Finished

You can revise a proposal forever, always finding little changes here and there. At some point you have to stop and begin the submission process. If the submission is late, you lose your opportunity!

Remember the Reader

Peer reviewers frequently have to read and score 10 or more proposals in a short period of time. Make it readable, interesting, and attention getting through picture words and active verbs.

process approach presented in this book will help you prepare and submit a complete, well-written, coherent, consistent, and supported proposal on time and within budget constraints.

This book uses a scaffolding approach to take you through the process with examples and practice so that writing a grant proposal becomes second nature for you. Once you have mastered the process, you will find that it can be used for other projects.

In the past, before grants were submitted electronically, one of my deans told me that *a proposal is never finished*; you can always find sections and sentences to edit for clarity, style, conciseness, and impact. However at some point you have to begin copying, collating, checking, and packaging for mailing. The same is true today; at some point before the deadline date and time the proposal has to be submitted for review. If you miss the deadline, you miss the opportunity to compete. If you are within an institution there are review steps leading up to final submission by your Office of Research and Sponsored Programs (ORSP) (a.k.a. grants office), and often your final proposal must be ready a week or more ahead of the actual deadline for review. Many times the final review process will reveal inconsistencies or errors you did not catch, and so it is equally important that you be available to consult on or complete any changes that need to be made before submission.

It is also critically important that the proposal be clear, readable, and understandable by those who review your submission. You will see that by using the exact headings provided in the RFP you will make your task and that of the readers easier. In addition the prose cannot be stilted. As with good writing in general the reader must be drawn in by your narrative. One way to do this is to use a suggestion I was given by a member of a writing team I worked with: use the active voice through **picture words and action verbs.** In Appendix A you will see tables that contain examples of these.

The process of grant writing can be broken down into steps. When these steps are followed in sequence a complete and competitive grant proposal is the result. The approach taken here is to map out the proposal using charts, tables, and diagrams and then to write the narrative that explains and supports what you are going to do.

A proposal is designed to market you and your program to individuals or government agencies that have money to support projects of interest. Your proposal document must convince readers/funders that:

- The group you are intending to serve is within their preferred population group;
- The individuals you are serving have sufficient need to warrant funding;
- Your program objectives are specific, measureable, attainable, realistic, and time oriented (SMART);
- The logic model for your proposal shows a clear and effective process;
- Your program activities will lead to the achievement of the program objectives;
- Your program design addresses the needs of the group/population you are going to serve;
- The design/activities of your program have merit given your presentation of relevant supporting research;
- You and your organization are well qualified and are, in fact, the best group to carry out the program because of past experience, location, purpose, or mission;
- The expertise of the project directors and staff assures program success;
- The environment in which the program will occur allocates sufficient space and support; and
- The proposed evaluation will demonstrate that your objectives have been met.

A critical question you might ask is "Why learn to write and submit grant proposals?" There are several reasons:

First, tax levy funding for student scholarships, community projects, after-school activities, enrichment programs for students, parent workshops, urban renewal, health initiatives, curriculum development, professional development, research, and innovative approaches has never been easy to get; recently, funds allocated for these critical activities has become virtually nonexistent. Local, state, and federal governments and private and corporate funders have always funded these types of programs, but many individuals have not tapped these resources. Now with tax funding shrinking as greater constraints are put on the available dollars, more and more individuals are turning to non-tax sources—such as grants—to support programs.

As more individuals turn to these resources it will become more difficult to win funds. Proposals will have to become more carefully thought out, structured, supported, and crafted to sell the funders on the value of your program and your ability to carry out your plan and achieve success. Some funding programs provide

What Is Tax Levy Funding?

Many organizations that seek grant funding obtain their basic operating expenses through federal, state, or local taxes. While the funding received may be sufficient for business as usual, it often does not allow for innovative approaches. Grant funds will permit an organization to try something new. If it produces expected outcomes, they can adopt it as usual practice.

continuing grant seekers additional points for prior experience (U.S. Department of Education TRIO programs are the most well-known example) so that new first-time proposers must achieve an almost perfect submission to receive funding.

Further, there are many funding streams available, and although there is some commonality among funders regarding how and what to submit for funding, each opportunity demands adherence to a unique set of guidelines for how, what, when, and where to submit. This book will give you the information you need to understand and respond to RFPs.

Second, a majority of community-based organizations and schools depend on allocations and donations from constituencies to carry out programs and to provide needed services. In troubling economic times the support often decreases, forcing cuts in programs, reduction in services to constituencies, or cutbacks in personnel.

Third, grant writing and preparation is a challenging and creative process entailing working with others to:

- Identify needs (program purpose and goals);
- Decide what you can and want to accomplish (program objectives);
- Develop a logic model that shows the relationships among inputs/ resources, activities, outputs, outcomes (short term and long term), and impact;
- Determine what can be done to address the needs and achieve the objectives (program design);
- Design an approach to implement the activities you select (program design and program management);
- Organize an approach to assess whether you have accomplished the objectives (program evaluation); and
- Explain how you will let others know about your program (program dissemination).

Fourth, it is critical that you use the selection criteria provided in the RFP to structure your proposal and that you respond to each element completely in order to maximize the points you will receive. Grants are awarded using the scores that are provided by a panel of readers. Definitely for federal grants, and in some state grants, there are usually three readers who independently score your proposal using the point values for each element of the selection criteria. The readers' total scores are averaged, and all proposals are ranked in score order. Funding begins with the highest scoring proposal and continues

What Are Selection Criteria?

Each RFP provides a set of questions that must be answered in detail in your proposal. These "selection criteria" are associated with point values and are used by reviewers to "score" your work. The better you respond to the selection criteria, the more points you receive and the more likely it is that you will receive funding.

down the ranked list until funding is exhausted. The higher your score, the more likely you will be in the funding band.

You can find funding in several ways:

- Review available RFPs, using the Forecast of Funding Opportunities or an online search program (such as Grants.gov, Pivot, or the Foundation Center search program—see suggestions in Chapter 5) to determine the funding opportunities that are/will be available;

- Subscribe to newsletters and e-mail alerts that provide information on newly announced RFPs;

- Develop an organizational database to identify areas for funding along with needs, goals, objectives, and assessments;

- Maintain an electronic database of past proposals (funded and unfunded) with reviewer ratings if available; or, best,

- Employ a combination of all of the above.

Fifth, an aspect of the process that is ongoing and crucial, and takes place outside of grant preparation, involves knowing your organization. It is widely agreed that self-knowledge is the key to advancing new programs. This aspect relates to the idea phase and is comprised of continuing identification of *organizational needs, best practices, innovative programs*, and *future directions*. At least two or three times per year a group of individuals from across your organization should to meet to review and add to lists of needs, practices, programs, and directions. These individuals should agree to look at current literature pertinent to your organization and review research relevant to these areas for your organization based on previous discussions. It is critical, as well, that meetings such as these take place in relation to a specific RFP, as well as within the preparation phase, but with a smaller, more focused group.

Sixth, many organizations have ongoing improvement projects in which teams of your colleagues meet to design more effective approaches to managing various aspects of the ongoing work. In addition, there are well-documented national challenges that can be cited to support the grant work of your organization, including readiness to learn, mathematical literacy, supporting English language learners, high school graduation, college readiness, college persistence, college graduation, and career readiness. There is also a national effort to increase preparation in Science, Technology, Engineering, and Mathematics (STEM), and many funders are asking that this be a focus of proposals.

Seventh, a grant proposal is a working document. You never finish it; you merely stop writing in time to meet the funding deadline. Programs can be funded by multiple sources—as long as each funder's resources are used to underwrite clearly different aspects of a project. One well-written proposal can be the foundation for grants in response to a number of different RFPs.

At the beginning of each chapter that addresses a section of the grant proposal, the selection criteria guiding your writing of that section will be presented. These selection criteria can be found in the application packet for the grant that is part of the RFP. My approach has always been to excerpt the selection criteria from the RFP and use them as the template for the table of contents and for the grant narrative.

Eighth, and finally, you and your organization can practice proactive or reactive grant writing. A proactive approach is one in which your organization consistently and systematically considers local needs, challenges, and opportunities and how they might be met through external funding. Perhaps there is already a group that meets regularly to plan for future needs and innovations, but I think this is unlikely. Many institutions are siloed, that is, opportunities for cross-conversations focused on the future are limited by the daily pressing issues. In contrast, a reactive approach responds to individual RFPs as they are released and then scrambles to find a relevant program initiative to include. As a grant writer for the past 35 years at my college I can attest to the efficacy of a proactive mind-set but have been able to participate in such efforts only a handful of times.

CHAPTER SUMMARY

The process approach to proposal writing focuses on a set of systematic, organized, and thoughtful methods to conceptualize, design, write, edit, and finalize a competitive set of documents to submit to a funder. This chapter reviews ways in which an institution or organization can find ideas for proposals. In addition, a series of questions is posed so that the user can determine whether his or her idea, the target population, research-based activities, organizational strengths and the location of the project meet the requirements of the funding agency. Finally, seven reasons why institutions and organizations should seek external funding are presented. These can be used to motivate others in your institution to support your efforts to seek funding. They include dwindling tax levy funds for needed support initiatives for underrepresented urban and rural students; lessening of individual donations to support extracurricular programing; the challenge of creating a proposal and receiving funding; the selection criteria to provide a way of viewing the capabilities of your institution and creating innovative approaches to meeting needs; the in-depth knowledge of an institution/organization needed to write a proposal; support for ongoing improvement and development efforts; the use of a proposal as a working document; and creation of an institutional mind-set for attending and responding to funding opportunities.

CHAPTER 2

Elements of the Planning Process

- How should I get ready for the planning process?

- What questions should I ask to determine if my proposal is right for a funder?

- How should I go about identifying a funding source?

- Why develop group consensus before writing a grant proposal?

- What are the steps I can follow to develop group consensus around a project?

- Should I use average ratings to illustrate consensus?

- What is SWOT analysis?

- How does a project differ from a program?

- How can I prove that my target group has high unmet needs?

- What is a jigsaw puzzle strategy and how can it help me determine need?

The planning process for seeking funding includes identifying needed programs and locating funding sources or locating funding sources and then realizing that one of your programs, or an item on your list of needed programs, meets the goals of the funder. It is a process of matching the program and the funding source. Another aspect involves seeing the possibilities for additional/ new funding within current programs.

It is also possible that a proposal written in response to a different RFP might be a jumping-off point for a new proposal. The accompanying sidebar illustrates how the extensive planning process for one competition, which was postponed, was used as the basis for a similar grant with a different focus.

It is important to note that funders want to realize their goals and objectives and "selling" your program to a potential funder is very similar to a marketing strategy. It is helpful to keep the following questions in mind when

Use a Well-Written Proposal for Different RFPs

A college recently prepared a Title V cooperative grant proposal to facilitate student transfer from 2-year colleges to 4-year colleges by simplifying enrollment and supporting success. After significant planning and drafting of the proposal, we found out that Title V would be funding down the slate from a previous year and so would not be accepting new proposals.

The college determined that there was another proposal opportunity through Hispanic-Serving Institutions in STEM (HSI-STEM) programs in which we could incorporate all of the previous work to facilitate student transfer from 2-year colleges to 4-year colleges by focusing the efforts on enrollment and support for success in STEM.

Applying for this proposal also incorporated components of a previous preproposal we had submitted for funding of a STEM initiative.

determining whether a particular funder would be interested in supporting your proposal.

- Why would a particular funder be interested in supporting your program?
- How does your program reflect the mission and goals of the funder's program?
- Why should your organization be chosen over another to run the program?
- What is it about the design of your program that makes it a logical choice?
- Is your program clearly presented so that individuals unfamiliar with what you propose can visualize your program?
- Is the program management and individual responsibility clear?
- Are the outcomes of what you propose clear?
- Do you have a well-organized evaluation plan to determine if the objectives of your project are met?
- Does your proposal follow the funder's guidelines and/or the reader selection criteria?
- Is the writing clear and unambiguous?

Identifying Funding Sources

Funding can come from many sources. Whole industries and publishing ventures are dedicated to letting people know where grants can be found. While government grants are unlikely to go unspent, there are many small grants that are not awarded because people don't know enough to ask about them or find them. There are publications that are helpful to grant seekers, but the most current and up-to-date information is available through the Internet. All information on finding funding through online resources is summarized in Appendix B so that the reader/user of this book can find all this information in one location.

Almost all government agencies, corporations, and private foundations that offer funding opportunities have websites that include extensive information and guidelines for proposals. In the tables at the end of Chapter 5, the major funders in each area are reviewed with information on how to navigate their websites and the types of programs they fund.

Online versions of most grant sources can be accessed through the Internet—some are free while others are only available for a fee or through education institutions.

Several weekly publications regularly list available and awarded grants. These include the *Chronicle of Higher Education,* now available on the Internet, and the *Chronicle of Philanthropy,* also available online. The resourceful Internet user can use search engines to find many sites that feature funding information. Another possibility is to search for programs similar in focus to yours and determine whether funding was obtained and where it was awarded.

Building Program Consensus before Writing the Proposal

There are various techniques that can be used to build consensus in large groups to identify potential programs and to focus disparate purposes and objectives on a smaller number of goals and objectives. One means of identifying potential program ideas is to review needs with members of your staff. There are several ways to accomplish this using a communication technique referred to as a *concourse* (from the Latin *concursus,* meaning "a running together," as when ideas run together in thought). The value of consensus is that it works creatively to include all persons making the decision. It is the most powerful decision process, as all members agree to the final decision. Consensus also gives everyone the power to have his or her voice heard, forces people to listen to each other, and answers their concerns instead of moving past them. The techniques presented here include the Delphi Technique, forced consensus, consensus by voting, and SWOT analysis.

Consensus can help develop the components of the proposal:

1. Who will be served by the grant?
2. What are their needs?
3. What outcomes need to be achieved?
4. What objectives meet the needs?
5. How are objectives linked to the outcomes?
6. What activities will assure achievement of outcomes?

7. What staff is needed to implement the project?

8. How will you know the outcomes are been achieved?

The Delphi Technique

The Delphi technique enables a group of individuals to achieve agreement and is characterized as a group communication process that enables all points of view to be considered. It is important that participants who have a vested interest in the project be invited to participate.

As preparation for using the Delphi technique, a group of individuals generates sample statements either individually or as members of a subgroup. An easy way to generate these statements is by having each individual or group complete 10 or more index cards (or Post-it notes), each containing one need to be met using external funding. In the case of an education grant various questions or focusing statements can be used to stimulate thinking among participants. These include:

- What characteristics would successful students share?
- What would an exemplary graduate of your school look like?
- What are the most pressing needs of your school?
- What challenges must students meet to be academically successful?
- What barriers hamper the learning and performance of students in math?
- How can we assure that 9th-graders are promoted to 10th grade?

Once the list of statements is finalized, each person ranks the statements from most characteristic of their viewpoint/belief to least characteristic of their viewpoint/belief. By using a disparate sample of individuals, including (for an educational issue) parents, teachers, administrators, students, school counselors, security staff, and school partners, it is possible to identify the most agreed-upon statements while preserving individual subjectivity.

Forced Consensus

This approach can lead to consensus, but it is constrained by having each individual post 10 responses, one person at a time, to create a grid with rows and columns where each column represents a unique idea and the rows contain ideas compatible with or related to the column topic. Thus, the first person would likely put all his cards in the first row, each card in a different column; the next person would place cards containing compatible ideas in a corresponding existing column and cards containing new ideas in new columns. Figures 2.1, 2.2, and 2.3 show how forced consensus works to provide a basis for determining the group perception of the needs of a particular population

Need 1 — Writing skills

Need 6 — Study skills

Need 1 — Few or no role models

Need 6 — Academically underprepared

Need 1 — Faculty unapproachable

Need 6 — Join campus organizations

Need 2 — Reading

Need 7 — Mentoring

Need 2 — Math skills

Need 7 — Academic support and how to get it

Need 2 — Parents/family not supportive

Need 7 — Understand financial aid and how to apply

Need 3 — College math

Need 8 — Academic advisement

Need 3 — Postponing required/prerequisite courses

Need 8 — Lack of confidence in ability

Need 3 — Balance work and school

Need 8 — Few resources to spend on college

Need 4 — Interact with teachers

Need 9 — Long-range planning

Need 4 — Critical thinking and problem solving

Need 9 — Feeling of isolation

Need 4 — Balance school and family

Need 9 — Work (for wages) takes priority

Need 5 — Computer skills

Need 10 — Time management skills

Need 5 — Comprehension skills

Need 10 — Unlikely to approach faculty

Need 5 — Not likely to see college as important

Need 10 — Technology skills

FIGURE 2.1. Examples of individual post-its.

Column 1	Column 2	Column 3	Column 4	Column 5	Column 6	Column 7
Need 1 Writing skills	Need 4 Interact with teachers	Need 8 Academic advisement	Need 7 Mentoring	Need 9 Long-range planning	Need 10 Time management skills	Need 10 Technology skills
Need 2 Reading	Need 10 Unlikely to approach faculty	Need 7 Understand financial aid and how to apply	Need 8 Lack of confidence in ability	Need 3 Postponing required/prerequisite courses	Need 3 Balance work and school	Need 5 Computer skills
Need 2 Math skills	Need 1 Faculty unapproachable	Need 6 Academically underprepared	Need 5 Not likely to see college as important	Need 8 Few resources to spend on college	Need 4 Balance school and family	
Need 3 College math		Need 7 Academic support and how to get it	Need 2 Parents/family not supportive		Need 9 Work (for wages) takes priority	
Need 5 Comprehension skills			Need 9 Feeling of isolation		Need 1 Few or no role models	
Need 4 Critical thinking and problem solving					Need 6 Join campus organizations	
Need 6 Academically underprepared						
Need 6 Study skills						

FIGURE 2.2. Post-its from Figure 2.1 organized into categories.

Column 1: Students are frequently underprepared for college work and may require assistance with mastering college-level mathematics (college algebra and precalculus), college-level writing (synthesis, editing, context, referencing), critical thinking and problem solving, quantitative reasoning, and reading/reading in the content areas (comprehension, vocabulary).

Column 2: Students are often reluctant to approach faculty members during office hours, as they see asking for help as a sign of weakness. This may be because of past experience. Students who work and have families often come onto campus for their courses and then spend little or no time because of external pressures. Finally, there are, unfortunately, a few faculty who actively discourage student inquiries.

Column 3: Students need early and frequent academic advisement to comprehend requirements, learn how to register for courses, understand the policies and procedures for financial aid, and appreciate the value of a long-range plan for prerequisites and corequisites and selection of a major.

Column 4: Students need to find or be assigned a mentor or coach or senior student or be in an affinity group of students with similar majors, areas of study, or interests who can guide them, without judgment, through the maze that is college for freshmen, and doubly confusing for first-generation college students, This is especially true for first generation students who often experience feelings of isolation.

Column 5: In order to complete college in 4–6 years students need a long-range plan and an understanding of prerequisites and corequisites. Students need to realize that a total of 30 credits a year or 15 per semester is needed to assure timely graduation. Students who have to work or raise families, especially, need a plan that includes summer and winter courses as well as online courses to keep them on track for graduation.

Column 6: First-generation students, especially those who work and have families to support or family responsibilities, need to be able to manage their time and finances so that they can effectively and efficiently complete necessary schoolwork and so they can plan finances to afford college completion. This may be especially critical for students who transfer from 2-year colleges as they are frequently in danger of running out of financial aid before completing their degree requirement.

Column 7: Although most students are familiar with smartphones, iPads, and social media, most cannot effectively use software applications or technology needed to manage online coursework. As many colleges now offer many required courses online, these students are at a disadvantage.

FIGURE 2.3. Summary of columns from Figure 2.2.

Achieving Consensus

More often than not grants are intended for institutionwide programs and projects. Therefore various decision makers have to be involved in shaping the proposal—particularly identifying goals, objectives, activities, and desired outcomes.

In the current funding climate, as well, there is a demand for interinstitutional collaboration by funding agencies. Interest has grown in 2-year/4-year college collaboration for transfer and BA completion; collaboration between high schools and colleges to facilitate access to and completion of college; collaboration between colleges and schools in teacher education; and collaboration between colleges and business/industry to prepare individuals for careers.

Use of a consensus process can give all participants an equal voice in shaping the project and will assure buy-in once funding is received.

of college students. Forms 1 and 2 are located at the end of the book and are downloadable for your use in a forced consensus process. The suggestions in the example are general, but the group might want to focus more narrowly by posing questions such as

- What are the needs of students enter nursing or allied health programs?
- What are the needs of students seeking degrees in STEM areas?
- What prerequisite experiences do students minoring in data science require?
- How can community college students be best prepared to transfer to senior colleges?
- How can college readiness be assured for high school students?

You might also want to use this approach to identify activities that will address the needs you have identified. For example:

- What activities would introduce students to and cultivate their interest in careers in nursing or teaching or STEM?
- What interventions would improve student writing ability?
- How can we assure that first-time freshmen are prepared for their college classes?
- What strategies will increase retention and graduation rates of first-generation students?

After all cards are placed, the group reviews the columns and judges whether any columns or cards should be combined. After those columns that are judged common in idea are combined, two individuals or groups each take a share of the columns and summarize the contents with a single statement. These statements then form the consensus of the group as to the most important needs. The statements that are generated can be used by the group to generate program ideas, project objectives, and/or activities. They can also be used to provide the items/statements/goals/purposes for the next approach.

Consensus by Voting

A simpler way to accomplish the same goal is to list items/statements/goals/ purposes on a chart or charts and provide individuals with sticky dots to use in identifying preferred items. These statements may be agreed upon by the group in discussion, culled from interviews with faculty, administrators, students or parents, or from previous procedures. After all have placed their dots, the items with the most dots are those that will be given priority. This process can be modified in various ways to provide a finer-grained analysis. Individuals can be provided with a fixed number of sticky dots and instructed to place one dot on each of their choices or to place one or more dots on fewer choices.

So, if we use the results of the forced consensus activity, each person would have seven dots. They can be the same color or different colors. Each person can place one or more dots as he or she chooses. The choice with the most dots would be given priority number one, the second most priority number two, and so on. Alternately, and for a larger group, the list could be printed out and individuals instructed to number all items in priority order from one to eight. The average ratings would be computed and the items ranked in order.

Another approach, helpful if different constituencies are represented, is to use dots of different colors to represent each constituency. For example, administrators might have one color, teachers another, students a third color, and parents a fourth color. Those items with the most votes would have priority, but it will be possible to differentiate among the represented constituencies to determine if there are similarities and differences among the groups. An example of this is shown in Table 2.1. (Only four respondents—represented by the letters A–D—are given, but any number may be surveyed. Survey Monkey can be used to facilitate administration of data to a large number of participants and analysis of it.)

SWOT Analysis

SWOT stands for *s*trengths and *w*eaknesses (internal factors) and *o*pportunities and *t*hreats (external factors). It is generally used to support strategic planning within institutions but can be helpful in preparing for grant seeking. It is designed to assist a group or organization to focus on key issues. You can develop the basic analysis in a brainstorming session. Some sample questions in each section may help you focus your group.

- **Strengths.** What does your institution/school/center do well? Some questions to help you get started are: What makes you stand out? What advantages do you have over others? How do your student outcomes differ from other institutions?
- **Weaknesses.** What do you struggle to accomplish? What do students/ parents/teachers complain about? What are the unmet needs of your students/teachers/administrators?

TABLE 2.1. Summary of Average Rankings Using Statements from Figure 2.2

	A	B	C	D	Average rank	Order based on ranking
Statement 1: Students are frequently underprepared for college work and may require assistance with mastering college-level skills.	1	2	3	2	2	2
Statement 2: Students are often reluctant to approach college faculty members during office hours, after class, by e-mail, or online.	2	3	1	3	2.25	3
Statement 3: Students need early and frequent academic advisement.	3	1	2	1	1.75	1
Statement 4: Students need to find (or be assigned) a mentor or coach who can guide and support them.	6	4	5	6	5.25	5
Statement 5: In order to complete college in 4–6 years, students need to have a long-range plan and understand the notion of prerequisites and corequisites.	4	5	4	5	4.5	4
Statement 6: First-generation students, especially those who work and have families or family responsibilities, need to be able to manage their time and finances	5	6	7	4	5.5	6
Statement 7: Too many students are not aware of the types of programs that can facilitate their work in college or help them manage online courses	7	7	6	7	6.75	7

Note. Each respondent ranks statements 1 through 7, where 1 is the top priority and 7 is the lowest. Rankings are then averaged. Statements from Figure 2.2 are used as the basis for individuals to rank the priority.

- **Opportunities.** What are some areas where your strengths are not being fully utilized? Are there emerging programs/materials/approaches that fit with your school's strengths? Is there a product/service that might be helpful but hasn't been adapted because of costs associated with implementation?

- **Threats.** Are your competitors becoming stronger? Are there emerging trends that will make one of your school's weaknesses especially damaging to student learning or school success? Do you see other external threats to student/teacher/school success? Internally, do you have financial, curriculum, supplies, materials, development, or other problems?

To begin the analysis, create a four-cell grid or four lists, one for each component: strengths, weaknesses, opportunities, and threats. These internal and external factors can be juxtaposed as seen in Table 2.2 to match strengths with opportunities. A blank SWOT analysis chart is provided in Form 3.

Use this information to develop programmatic areas and specific activities that would strengthen the organization, motivate teachers, increase student

TABLE 2.2. Summary of SWOT Components

	Internal	External
Positive	**Strengths** What are the internal strengths of the organization/program/office? Determine how the organization can overcome poor outcomes by using its strengths to prevent unmet needs from undermining outcomes.	**Opportunities** What are the strengths of the organization/program/office as it relates to the external community? Use organizational strength to pursue opportunities that fit well with what the organization does well.
Negative	**Weaknesses** What are the internal weaknesses of the organization/program/office? Develop strategies to use opportunities to overcome identified weaknesses (needs) in terms of educational outcomes.	**Threats** Weaknesses can leave an organization vulnerable to external factors. How can funding assist in overcoming weaknesses to meet targets or mitigate the impact of threats?

outcomes, and raise the level of accomplishment of the school. Then match funding opportunities with your desired outcomes.

Wish Lists

Wish lists are a more informal method. Individuals in your organization are asked to develop wish lists—What do you want to happen differently? How do you want students to perform? What would you need to have a model school with ideal outcomes for all students? What if you had $50,000 to spend on changing something you are doing or that the school is doing? A consensus procedure can also be used once a project area has been developed to focus and refine the idea. Focus groups can be used to explore reactions to ways to address organizational needs that have been identified and projects that might be developed to resolve them. It should also be noted that there are many online survey programs (e.g. Survey Monkey, Zoomerang, Snap, Qualtrics Insight Platform, and Polldaddy) that can be used to elicit feedback or input from individuals in a computer-based form.

Moving from Project to Program Approach

Another approach to identifying opportunities for increased funding is to look at your institution/district/center in terms of programs, not projects. A project, by definition, has a defined beginning and a defined end with specific goals and objectives. When they are attained the project is viewed as completed. A programmatic approach, by contrast, is a set or group of coordinated efforts that together or sequentially build upon one another to obtain outcomes and results that are more far-reaching than what one isolated project can accomplish. Table 2.3 clarifies the differences between a project and a program.

In order to successfully accomplish a project you need input from a small number of individuals and a set of circumscribed goals and objectives. For a successful program you must develop a philosophy that relates to the location of the institution, its needs, the population it serves, national reports, whole schools, feeder patterns, and collaboration. Other factors include the following: Are the institutions urban, suburban, or rural? How far are the participants to be served from the host institution? How will the participants get to the host institution, or will the host institution carry the program to them?

For example, an urban college is embarking on a 12-year effort to double the number of degrees and certificates it awards (in comparison to the number anticipated within that time with no changes). In order to accomplish this, the

TABLE 2.3. Differences between Project and Program

	Project	Program
Objectives	Outputs—tangible; relatively easy to describe, define, and measure; tending toward objective.	Outcomes—often intangible; difficult to quantify; benefits often based on changes to organizational culture/behaviors; introducing new capabilities into the organization; tending toward subjective.
Scope	Strictly limited; tightly defined; not likely to be subject to change during the life of the project.	Not tightly defined or bounded; likely to change during the life cycle of the program.
Duration	Relatively short term; typically 3 to 6 months.	Relatively long term typically 18 months to 3 years.
Risk profile	Project risk is relatively easy to identify and manage. The project failure would result in relatively limited impact on the organization relative to program risk.	Program risk more complex and potential impact on the organization if a risk materializes will be greater relative to project risk. Program failure could result in material financial, reputational, or operational loss.
Nature of the problem	Clearly defined.	Ill defined; often disagreement among key stakeholders on the nature/definition of the problem.
Nature of the solution	A relatively limited number of potential solutions.	Significant number of potential solutions, often with disagreement between stakeholders as to the preferred solution.
Stakeholders	A relatively limited number of stakeholders.	A significant number of diverse stakeholders; probable disagreement as to the definition of the problem and preferred solution.
Relationship to environment	Environment within which the project takes place is understood and relatively stable.	Environment is dynamic; program objectives need to be managed in the context of the changing environment within which the organization operates.
Resources	Resources to deliver the project can be reasonably estimated in advance.	Resources are constrained and limited; there is competition for resources between projects.

Note. Reprinted with permission from **www.independent-consulting-bootcamp.com.**

college must define its philosophy with respect to growing admission, supporting students, enhancing persistence, increasing retention, and facilitating transfer of students; the college must analyze location of the institution and develop a profile of current, entering, and potential students to be served; and as the urban college enrollment may be impacted by the K–12 system in its community, the college must study the current and expected student achievement to determine future potential for enrollment. The reality is that the potential high school graduates in our community should now be in preschool and will enter kindergarten in September 2018. The college graduates of 2030 are currently in 4th grade and will be entering 5th grade in September 2018. In order to achieve its goal the urban college will have to include a significant outreach effort to the schools and communities in its locale.

Showing Need

The most critical aspect of the grant development process is establishing need. In order to prepare a competitive needs section, you should use demographic data including data on ethnicity, income, education, poverty levels, and employment.

School data are also helpful in establishing need for different approaches. This can include graduation rates, high school cohort progress, attendance rates, standardized test scores, college application rates, enrollment in 2- and 4-year colleges, transfer rates from 2- to 4-year colleges, performance in gateway courses, GPAs and time to BA completion.

The most critical aspect of any program is need. What are the needs of the host institution, of participants, of the education system, and of the individual schools? There are many ways to discover this, and I would recommend developing a comprehensive needs statement using local, state, and national reports on educational status and outcomes. Census reports for any state, city, or zip code using American FactFinder provide a range of information. The link is **https://factfinder.census.gov/faces/nav/jsf/pages/index.xhtml.** The reports provide population data for categories including age, business and industry, education, governments, housing, income, origins and language, poverty, race and Hispanic status, and veteran status. In addition, local, city, and state governments issue economic reports as well as information on health issues and concerns and employment status. Time spent in developing extensive data on need will serve you well in the long run, as establishing need is a critical component of any grants you will prepare. Often community organizations at the local, state, and national levels publish regular reports on a wide variety of topics related to need.

An example from American FactFinder is shown in Table 2.4. When you open American Factfinder, you will find the webpage shown in Figure 2.4. Please note that a blank form for your use is at the end of the book and available for download.

Type in your city and state or zip code in the space provided and hit "GO." You will see the content presented in Figure 2.5.

You want to select a category from the left side list. I selected education and then selected "Educational attainment" to get the data for Table 2.4.

In order to use these data in your proposal, you would want to extract and create tables for the specific information relevant to your goal and objectives. Form 4, located at the end of the book, is downloadable and can be used for your own data presentation. The community in which most of my grants

TABLE 2.4. Example of Educational Attainment for the United States in 2016

Category	Total % estimate	Males % estimate	Females % estimate
Population 25 years and over			
Less than 9th grade	5.6%	5.7%	5.4%
9th–12th grade, no diploma	7.4%	8.0%	6.9%
High school graduate (includes equivalency)	27.5%	28.2%	26.9%
Some college, no degree	21.0%	20.6%	21.2%
Associate degree	8.2%	7.3%	9.0%
Bachelor's degree	18.8%	18.6%	19.0%
Graduate or professional degree	11.5%	11.5%	11.5%
Population 25 to 34 years			
High school graduate or higher	89.3%	87.7%	90.9%
Bachelor's degree or higher	33.7%	29.7%	37.8%
Race and Hispanic or Latino Origin			
White alone, not Hispanic or Latino			
High school graduate or higher	92.0%	91.5%	92.5%
Bachelor's degree or higher	33.8%	34.2%	33.5%
Black			
High school graduate or higher	84.3%	82.9%	85.6%
Bachelor's degree or higher	20.0%	17.4%	22.2%
American Indian/Alaska Native			
High school graduate or higher	79.3%	77.6%	81.0%
Bachelor's degree or higher	14.0%	12.8%	15.2%
Asian			
High school graduate or higher	86.3%	88.2%	84.6%
Bachelor's degree or higher	52.1%	54.7%	49.8%
Native Hawaiian/Other Pacific Islander			
High school graduate or higher	86.4%	86.7%	86.1%
Bachelor's degree or higher	16.2%	16.0%	16.4%
Hispanic or Latino Origin			
High school graduate or higher	65.7%	64.2%	67.2%
Bachelor's degree or higher	14.7%	13.4%	16.1%

(continued)

TABLE 2.4. *(continued)*

Category	Total % estimate	Males % estimate	Females % estimate
Poverty rate			
Less than high school graduate	27.1%	23.3%	30.9%
High school graduate (includes equivalency)	14.3%	12.2%	16.3%
Some college or Associate degree	10.4%	8.3%	12.3%
Bachelor's degree or higher	4.5%	4.1%	4.9%

Note. Margin of error = 0.1–0.2. Data from **https://factfinder.census.gov/faces/nav/jsf/pages/index.xhtml**.

are located is majority Hispanic/Latino origin. The table shows that bachelor's degree or higher educational attainment for my population across the United States is 14.7%. This is a bit higher than my specific population. It also shows that the poverty rate for those 25 and over with a bachelor's degree is 4.5% contrasted with much higher poverty rates as educational attainment decreases. Thus, perhaps our goal of doubling the number of degrees and certificates in the next 12 years is a significant goal and critical for the growth of our community.

Funders want to know that you have done your homework and that you will employ approaches and activities that have the greatest chance of success. What does national research indicate? What activities and approaches have been successful with participants in the past? What data/evaluations do you have to show that your initiatives have been successful? How will you work with schools? Will you collaborate or form partnerships with whole schools or

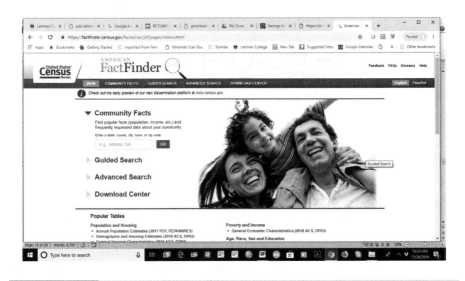

FIGURE 2.4. Screenshot of the American Fact Finder home page.

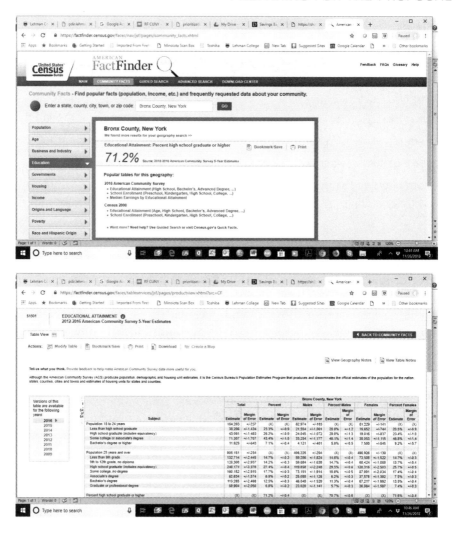

FIGURE 2.5. Screenshots of the opening view of the Bronx County, New York home page and the detail page for educational attainment.

systems or recruit students from a range of schools and systems? What approach would assure best use of time and resources?

In planning a comprehensive approach will you establish a farm–system model? Participants who begin in your program as middle school students will be encouraged to continue throughout high school and to maintain a connection (by assisting younger students) as they complete college. Many programs currently funded through the U.S. Department of Education (Upward Bound, Talent Search, GEAR UP) require that student participation be maintained through high school graduation and beyond and mandated evaluation criteria and objectives use high school graduation, college admission, and college entrance data to evaluate programs for continued funding. Do you have different programs that serve students at different education levels? Is there an approach that provides for students to move from one program to another? Do you have programs that offer different services so that participants can be served across programs? Can your programs be characterized using a pipeline model that encourages students to maintain connections with your institution throughout levels of education?

The Jigsaw Puzzle Strategy

Another approach to envisioning a programmatic approach is to see the projects you already have as part of a whole, a jigsaw puzzle if you like, in which the philosophy is the glue and with which all projects are potentially related. You must see the big picture and identify sections of the puzzle. Do you have projects that address ESL, professional development, school-to-work, basic skills, or parenting? Can the projects be related by population served, outcome desired, or thematic area? This is a time-consuming and cumbersome task in which you need to see the whole picture. One way to accomplish this is to create a table that includes projects under your purview. A sample table might look like the one presented in Table 2.5. A blank project overview chart is provided in Form 5.

The next step is to determine what elements are missing. What pieces are needed to complete the picture? Most funders would much prefer to contribute to a grand scheme than to support a single, unconnected project. Figure 2.6 illustrates a series of programs in mathematics and science that serve children in K—PhD. All these programs have been in place at one time or another, and the goal has been to encourage students to move from one level to the next as they progress in school. At one point all of the programs were in place except the Hughes Biological Sciences Program. We argued in our funding proposal that a "puzzle piece" filling in the space from 11th grade to college sophomore would encourage students to choose science majors in college and would bridge the high school/college science gap. We were funded. Further information regarding expansion of funding sources is presented in Figure 2.7.

Matching Programs and Funding

Each funding agency has priorities for what it wants to fund. The grant proposal has to demonstrate that the program has elements that can meet the priorities. This is a marketing strategy. You determine the needs of the market/funder and then emphasize those aspects of your product/program that best meet its needs. Think about the advertisements you see on TV or hear on the radio. They target a listener or viewer with specific needs (for a medicine) and then show how their medicine addresses that identified need. You will identify the needs of your community/population/school/college/students and show, based on best practices research and references, how your intended intervention/program will resolve the needs and improve outcomes.

TABLE 2.5. Overview of Projects

Grant	Goal	Objectives	Population	Activities	Outcomes
A	Increased promotion rates from 9th to 10th grade	• Incoming 9th graders better prepared for high school work • Pass rates in coursework increase • Homework completion increases • Attendance increases • Higher rates of promotion to 10th grade	Middle to high school transition students in urban schools	• Summer bridge to high school program • Orientation to high school • Content-based academic skills improvement • 9th-grade Saturday Academy	• Pass rates, grades, and promotion increase as compared to students who did not attend summer bridge or Saturday Academy program.
B	Improved reading for learning	• Increase student comprehension and synthesis • Increase student academic vocabulary • Improve student understanding of graphic symbols	Urban middle school students (monolingual and bilingual)	• Fluency First program • Use of reading guides for subject-based texts • Computer-based diagnostics • Use of didactic journals	• Pass rates, grades, and reading comprehension increase as compared to previous work • Individualize support.
C	Increased interest in STEM	• Improve mathematics skills • Increase readiness for algebra • Provide after-school tutoring • Improve understanding of science • Increase students' understanding of and engagement in research	Urban middle and high school students	• Math games • Use of manipulatives • Computer-based diagnostics • Hands-on science project	• Increased scores in math skills tests. Students report increased confidence with mathematics. • Higher mathematics grades
D	College readiness and access	• Dual enrollment programs • SAT/English/math modules • Summer college academies	Urban high school students	• Hands-on science project • Writing research reports • Computer programming	• Increased college readiness • Higher grades • Improved report writing

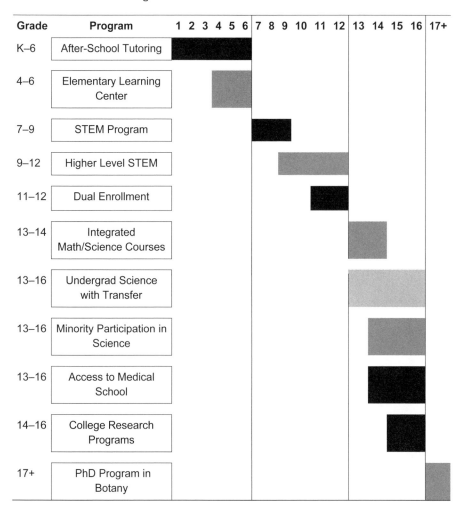

Grade	Program	1 2 3 4 5 6	7 8 9 10 11 12	13 14 15 16	17+
K–6	After-School Tutoring	██████			
4–6	Elementary Learning Center	▒▒▒			
7–9	STEM Program		███		
9–12	Higher Level STEM		▒▒▒▒		
11–12	Dual Enrollment		███		
13–14	Integrated Math/Science Courses			▒▒	
13–16	Undergrad Science with Transfer			░░░░	
13–16	Minority Participation in Science			▒▒▒	
13–16	Access to Medical School			███	
14–16	College Research Programs			██	
17+	PhD Program in Botany				▒

FIGURE 2.6. K–PhD science–mathematics linkages.

Using Figure 2.7, visualize a project/program as being in the center of the circle. Each segment represents a different funding source. Each source is seeking to fund a slightly different project. This is a marketing problem. How can you present your project in such a way that funding source 1, for example, sees it as a program that would be appropriate for agency 1 to fund? By emphasizing a slightly different need or aspect of your project can you "sell" funding source 2 on your program by making it seem to precisely meet agency 2 funding priorities? For example, suppose you are working with an urban school district to prepare students to enter STEM majors. Putting the program at the center of the circle and looking at it as an objective observer may suggest a number of differentiated aspects that could be developed for funding. Multiple sources of funding are permitted as long as different funding is not used for the same purpose.

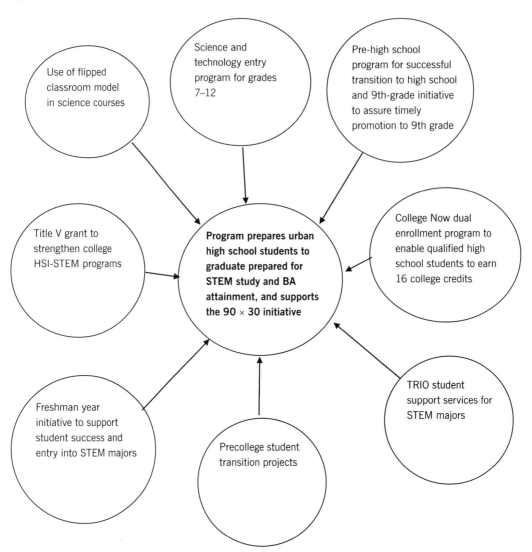

FIGURE 2.7. Organizing individual projects to achieve central program goals. 90 × 30 is an initiative at Lehman College in the Bronx, New York, aimed at granting 90,000 degrees and certificates by 2030.

So, let's use as an overall sample program goal increasing the number of underrepresented high school students who graduate from high school, are interested in STEM areas, qualify for college entrance, and are supported to graduate with a baccalaureate in a STEM area. We can see this as a pipeline/ college access issue that would appeal to funders who want to (1) increase the number of urban high school students involved in and prepared for success in STEM; (2) support 8th-grade students to prepare for the often difficult transition to high school; (3) support students during the freshman year in high school; (4) increase the number of urban high school students who, through

dual enrollment programs, complete college credits before high school graduation; (5) support urban students as they enter college; (6) provide opportuni-
ties/support for urban students to obtain high grades in gateway courses needed
to enter STEM majors; (7) strengthen urban/minority-serving institutions'
academic, fiscal, and management operations to better serve students; and (8)
develop innovative ways of teaching often difficult STEM courses with high
failure rates.

Expanding Funding

Using the model shown to match your program to the priorities of multiple
funders makes it easy to visualize the next step, that of obtaining funding for
the different aspects of your program from different sources. *This is entirely permissible so long as the funds from different sources are not used to fund the same activities.*
Different funders/funds could be used to support students at different grade
levels; support children and their parents; offer academic and sports classes;
replicate a successful program with children having different needs; or begin
with pre-K students and continue grade by grade through graduation from
college. Initially, you might review the current projects in your district and
determine whether additional funding could be obtained for any of the existing
projects if they were expanded to other schools, developed into magnet school
programs, recast as collaborations with other districts or colleges, designed to
address specific populations of students, focused on bringing the community
into the schools, or collaborations with business or industry, or designed to
extend successful programs districtwide.

Projects can also be linked into an overall program by seeking funding for
a program that includes such components as:

- *Academic content areas*—math, science, literacy, social studies, languages,
  and ELA (English language arts);
- *Counseling*—personal, academic, social, and college counseling;
- *After-school activities*—academic, recreation, mentoring, and sports;
- *Professional development for teachers*—curriculum, teaching, teacher men-
  toring, and planning;
- *Technology*—Internet, curriculum planning, computer equipment,
  school website, and e-mail;
- *Parent support*—computer literacy, family math/science, and financial
  aid assistance for college;
- *Student support*—thematic career education, tutoring, and mentoring;
  and
- *School resources*—classroom libraries, classroom technology, wireless
  Internet, and attendance systems.

There is an extensive array of areas to consider in designing and expanding programs. Grants are available to fund education programs in areas such as:

Academic Achievement	Leadership Development
Adolescent Health	Literacy Education
Adolescent Parenting	Mathematics Education
Adolescents	Minority Education
Alternative Education	Parent Education
At-Risk Students	Parent Involvement
Basic Skills Education	Precollege Education
Bilingual–Bicultural Education	Preschool Education
Career Education and Planning	Professional Development
Community and School Partnerships	Promise Neighborhoods
Community Health	Science Education
Continuing Education	Special Education
Cooperative Education	Speech and Hearing
Dropout Prevention	STEAM
Education and Work	STEM
Educational Evaluation	Student Enrichment
Educational Technology	Students with Disabilities
Educational Reform	Teacher Attitudes
Gifted and Talented	Teacher Education
Health Education	Urban Education
Journalism	Youth Development/Leadership

CHAPTER SUMMARY

Elements of the planning process highlight the tasks that are central to the exploration and development of potential projects that will serve your institution/organization. Projects or needs that have been identified can be matched to available funding, or projects can be developed in response to available funding announcements. Emphasis is on the notion of "marketing" your idea to the funder. How does your idea contribute to the mission, vision, or purposes of the funder? Assuming that you have a project idea, how do you go about finding funding that will support your goals and objectives? In the planning for a proposal it is helpful to achieve organizational consensus. Several procedures for engaging groups of individuals and synthesizing their input are presented with examples of the process. Many institutions/organizations can effectively link projects that serve multiple constituencies and needs but must consider the differences between a single project approach and a program approach before proceeding. This chapter also highlights the critical importance of establishing/proving need. Finally, the process of linking projects and matching projects to funding sources is presented.

CHAPTER 3

Collaborative and Interdisciplinary Approaches

LEARNING OBJECTIVES

- Why collaborate with other institutions/individuals?

- Why is a long-term approach to identifying grant possibilities a good idea?

- What is a collaborative grant-writing continuum?

- How can each partner in a collaboration feel equal?

While collaboration and interdisciplinary approaches have been encouraged for some time, over the past decade they have become two of the most mandated approaches suggested in RFPs and, in fact, sometimes constitute a section that is associated with scoring criteria. Both approaches require working with other institutions, departments, disciplines, and people and necessitate allocating longer planning time, more reviews of the proposal, lengthy discussions about budgets, decisions about finances, agreements on who will be the lead partner, and preparation of memoranda of understanding (partnership agreements, contracts, and subcontracts). All of these mean that planning and writing must start well in advance of the deadline date. Given that most federal grant announcements are released only 30–45 days before the due date, institutions/grant writers need to develop proposal frameworks that emphasize collaboration and interdisciplinary approaches regularly to address the needs of the institution and its partners. Since most RFPs are somewhat consistent from competition to competition, last year's outline can be used to begin the planning and collaboration process well in advance of official announcements.

Fortunately, all of the strategies presented in Chapter 2 can be used to facilitate collaboration between and among institutions, departments, or disciplines. Often the most difficult problem to be overcome is to have the final proposal look like a cohesive, well-organized, focused plan rather than a document that resulted from too many cooks. In my grant-writing experience I have been involved in writing collaborative/partnership proposals of both types. Most recently, three were submitted and only one was funded. I believe that of the three, two used processes that were successful in creating a cohesive collaborative program. Let me share the effective strategies that led to successful collaborations. Dopke and Crawley (2013) have suggested that effective groups use strategies related to small-group decision making. They further suggest that shared writing presents a difficult dynamic and can be problematic; this is why I suggest that writing be assigned to one or, at most, two designated individuals. The points below are also presented graphically in Figure 3.1, which will enable the reader to visualize the progress of collaboration.

1. Partners/collaborators must be identified and approached early (a year ahead of an anticipated deadline)

2. Representatives (henceforth referred to as the "team") should be designated by each institution, have equal status within their institutions, and have the power to make decisions. Care must be taken to designate individuals who have the skills to work collaboratively and the institutional knowledge required to make good choices.

3. The team should tentatively designate the "lead institution" that will serve as the fiscal agent for the grant, and the ORSP of that institution will assist in creating a budget for the project, which will be shared with all other collaborating institutions for input and review.

4. Joint needs, goals, and objectives should be determined through a lengthy brainstorming session with detailed notes.

5. Notes should be transcribed verbatim and circulated to the team for review, comments, and corrections.

6. Team members, at the next meeting, will prioritize the needs, goals, and objectives.

7. The lead writer (designated by the group) or cowriters (one from each institution), designated as "grant writer(s)," will provide a set of table templates for each institution to use in identifying the needs of its population and to summarize best practices currently being implemented.

8. The grant writers will use the material provided by each institution to draft a needs section for the proposal.

9. Team members will review the section and provide corrections, comments, and general feedback.

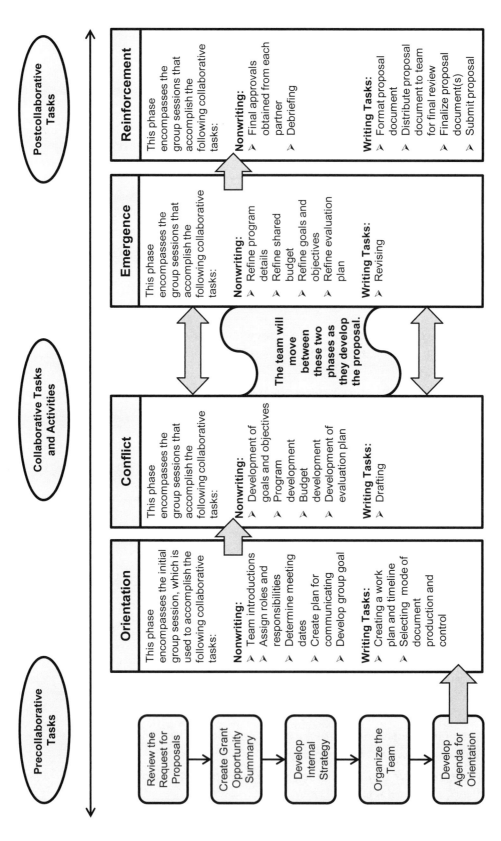

FIGURE 3.1. Collaborative grant-writing continuum. From Dobke and Crawley (2013). Copyright © 2013 Society of Research Administrators International. Reprinted by permission.

34

As the proposal development proceeds, Steps 4–9 should be followed to draft each section of the proposal. Through this process the proposal should be ready in draft form well before the RFP is released. The draft proposal should be reviewed within each institution and approved for further development once the actual RFP is released. Once this occurs, the grant writers will review the proposal, highlight needed changes related to the RFP, use Track Changes to make them, and circulate a draft to the team for review, comment, correction, and approval.

Once the proposal is in final form, it should be reviewed by each collaborating partner and approved for submission. The lead institution/fiscal agent will be responsible for submitting the proposal, ideally before the actual deadline.

CHAPTER SUMMARY

In the current funding climate, partnerships and collaborations are frequently emphasized. Accordingly, this chapter addresses some critical considerations in partnering with other institutions and organizations. Use of a logic model, discussed more fully in Chapter 9, will facilitate collaboration among partners.

CHAPTER 4

Broadening, then Focusing, Your Project

LEARNING OBJECTIVES

- What questions need to be answered before conceptualizing a project?

- How can I find community stakeholders?

- Why should my institution/ organization maintain a database of program connections?

- Are there characteristics of my institution that might qualify me for special grants?

- What questions do I need to ask to go from a broad to a focused approach?

- Why should I think of my project as a marketing effort?

There are two ways to approach creating a grant proposal: the first is to have an RFP that seems to fit your organization and some of its needs or priorities and to develop your idea into a proposal using the goals, objectives, guidelines, and selection criteria of the RFP; the second is to develop a project that would strengthen your organization or the partnership you are working in, seek an RFP that will fund your project, and then develop your idea into a proposal. In the areas to be discussed in this chapter an initial broader view will assist you to conceptualize your final submission to the funding source or to the RFP.

Either way, as conveyed by the title of this chapter, the first conceptualization of your project should be as broad and far-reaching as the context, mission, and vision for the proposal you will develop and finally submit. You need to answer one or more of these overall questions:

- What should a participant in this project know and be able to do as a result of involvement?

- What will my school be able to accomplish for its students as a result of this project?

- How will my institution be better as a consequence of putting this program in place?
- How will this project help my institution and its students address the needs we have identified?

Determining the Scope and Direction of Your Project

The first task in conceptualizing the scope and direction of your project is to identify potential stakeholders within your organization or community. Rarely is a proposal the work of a single person, and you should use one of the consensus processes identified in Chapter 2 to assure input from the individuals who will be impacted/assisted by the project to be implemented.

Every institution or organization is part of a larger local, regional, state, or national community. If the broad approach to your proposal can address broad issues/concerns/problems by finding solutions that address your institution/organization, your arguments for sustainability and dissemination will be enhanced. Your organization likely has many connections already but probably not a comprehensive list of contacts and missions. Several years ago my college created a school/college collaborative directory that summarized all of the partnerships/agreements our institution had with schools and school-related agencies in our city. We used to publish paper copies each year and distribute them. Unfortunately, we failed to maintain the database as an online resource for the future, and so we lost an important source of information. For lack of a database such as this, members of our institution are often surprised to find, when approaching a new partner, that the college already has a program connection there.

The SWOT process can lead to identification of strengths and weaknesses and can produce ideas for a project that will capitalize on the strengths while addressing the weaknesses. Alternately a project can use strategies that will focus on ameliorating the weaknesses while using the strengths to support new initiatives.

Another approach is to look at a profile of your institution and determine whether it falls into one or more specific areas targeted for funding by various agencies reviewed in Chapter 5. For example, there has recently been recognition that low-income, first-generation students who are also Black or Hispanic achieve baccalaureate degrees at a percentage far below their representation in the population. For many years there have been RFPs focused on improving preparation and graduation rates for students at historically Black colleges and universities (HBCU). Recently focus has turned to Hispanic-serving institutions (HSIs) and minority-serving institutions (MSIs), and many RFPs seek to serve individuals in these institutions. In the case of targeted RFPs, the institution has to use a two-step process by first seeking certification as an HIS/MSI and, once it is received, submitting a proposal. You need to have a broad view of the project in terms of the following:

- Why is your organization qualified or equipped to conduct this project?
- Who should be targeted?
- What are their needs?
- How will participants be identified?
- What will participants be able to do as a result of the project that they cannot do now?
- Will the project be located within or outside of your organization?
- Will there be partners and/or collaborators?
- When will the project begin and what are the assessment points for evaluation and modification?
- How will the project relate to the current structure of your organization?

You will use this information in two different ways: first to broaden and then sharpen your project by searching the research literature to determine what interventions and strategies have been shown to work for your students, your institution, and your community. Increasingly, funders want to assure that the project activities to be implemented have been shown to be effective. Over the past 5–10 years RFPs have included competitive priorities that earn additional points when supported by research findings that have been verified through the Institute of Education Sciences What Works Clearinghouse (WWC). Once you have this information, you can determine what funders are willing to support and/or consider the types of projects that are being funded and can begin to list project topics and emphases. Often when searching for funding I use broad keywords and leave my mind open to the range of possibilities that might present themselves. Your goal is to determine the types of projects that are being funded or that are sought by funding agencies and foundations. If you are at an educational institution, you may have access to a variety of funding databases. All the information in this book related to online resources for searching funding databases and specific funding agencies, corporations, and foundations is provided in Chapter 5.

Matching Your Proposal to the Funding Guidelines

You may now have a broadly conceived notion of the content area of your proposal or a more focused idea with related objectives, activities, and desired outcomes. You (and your team) must now make a critical shift and shape your idea according to the guidelines and language of the proposal. Most federal RFPs now contain a section entitled "Performance Measures." These are the guidelines for project evaluation and program success. For example:

> The success of the UBMS Program will be measured by the percentage of UBMS participants who enroll in and complete postsecondary education. (*Federal Register,* Vol. 82, No. 27, Friday, February 10, 2017, p. 10353)

The set of performance measures includes specific course enrollment, graduation, college enrollment, placement in college-level courses, AA or BA degree attainment in timely fashion, completion of Free Application for Federal Student Aid (FAFSA), and cost per participant. Your program design, including objectives, activities, and personnel, must be focused on achieving these outcomes. Frequently, RFPs indicate required, permissible, and nonpermissible activities that can be used to achieve the goals and objectives of the project. This information will enable you to begin to narrow your choices.

You might want to use a version of the consensus process and have individuals use sticky notes to identify (1) project goals; (2) hurdles preventing the target population from reaching them; (3) objectives that move participants toward the goal; (4) activities that will enable objectives to be attained; (5) expected outcomes; (6) who will guide the activities; (7) how you will determine (measure) that the objective is achieved; (8) how much it will cost; and (9) what the impact will be.

Sorting and comparing the notes at each step and using the group consensus at each step to inform the next will result in a fairly robust set of entries for a preliminary table. A useful model for me has always been to create a table, as the rows and columns correspond to the headings that will be needed for the final narrative. So the overall title of your table is one of goals you wish to achieve through your project, the rows are the objectives developed to realize the goal, and the columns are the activities, outcomes, personnel, timeline, and measures that will enable you to attain the objectives and the related goal (see Table 4.1). This table will also enable you to create the logic model needed to test the connectedness of the proposal.

Deconstructing Your Project

Now that you have a table with the elements that drive the narrative for your project, the next step is to determine what you know and what information is needed to support the activities and their value to achieving the objectives of the project. In particular, is there moderate evidence from research to support the expected outcomes of the activities you will implement? Can you cite research, particularly research vetted by the Institute of Education Sciences and presented in the WWC, that will support the activities you propose?

TABLE 4.1. Program Goal 1: Improve College Readiness, Access, and Completion for Students Who Have Been Traditionally Underrepresented in Postsecondary Education

Need	Objective	Activity	Outcome	Personnel	Measure	Budget	Impact
Financial aid	Increase the percentage of students who complete the online FAFSA by 5% each year	Parent workshops; student FAFSA sessions; texted student reminders	Parents understand importance; students complete FAFSA	Financial aid personnel; financial counselor; student advisers	No. and percentage of students completing FAFSA from year to year		More parents and students aware of and receiving financial support
Standardized test-taking skills	Increase the average SAT scores of students by 80 points	SAT preparation workshop with concurrent English class	Students obtain higher scores from pre- to posttest	External SAT preparation firm; college instructor	Pre–post comparison of average SAT scores and improvement	$7,000 per preparation class ($N = 20$); $3,500 for English instructor	More students are eligible to enter 4-year colleges

Marketing Your Project

A grant proposal is similar to a marketing campaign. You are selling yourself and your institution as the best choice for achieving the outcomes that the funder wants. The proposal needs to tell a story of how the participants will be changed for the better and will be able to achieve the overall goal of the project by being served by your project. You need to answer the following questions:

- Why will you be successful?
- How will you engage the students to persist in your project?
- What will you do to encourage them to do their best work?
- What are the skills and strengths of you and your institution that set you apart and qualify you for funding?

Your excitement and belief in what you will be able to accomplish have to come through early in your narrative. You have to capture the readers' interest within the first two pages. Your project has to matter in the lives of those you will serve.

Choosing the Most Appropriate Funding Opportunity

If you find that there are several seemingly appropriate funding opportunities that fit your proposed project, you may want to consider some additional factors in choosing the one that best fits your institution. Consider the following:

- Does the RFP mention that prior grantees receive extra points, sometimes called prior experience points?
- Is the funding offered by the RFP sufficient for you to employ the staff you need to be successful?
- How well does your institution fit the profile for funding consideration?
- For how long is the funding provided?
- Can/does your institution comply with all of the rules and regulations of the funder?

Multiple Proposals to Support the Same Project

Figure 2.5 in Chapter 2 can be used as a way to identify funders for different aspects of a single project or to identify various projects that would fit into a larger programmatic concept. In this instance it is used to focus your attention on the fact that a funder may only be interested in supporting a particular narrow aspect of your project, such as student services, but you believe that teacher development is an important part of the changes you are seeking to make. So you can change the focus of your project and submit it to a funder who will support the additional focus. As indicated previously it is crucial that funds do not overlap. Figure 4.1a is a template in which you identify a program goal and then view it from many perspectives to see if funders might want to focus on different aspects. Figure 4.1b shows a completed version with a program goal and several funders whose RFPs suggest that they would want to fund various aspects of the program.

Another problem is that if you seek to share positions between or among grants, a full salary can be dependent on getting all grants funded. This does not always happen. Many times the easiest positions to share are the administrative assistants, data analysts, student assistants, and secretary/receptionists.

Figure 4.1a (and the completed version presented in Figure 4.1b) can be useful in exploring how **different funders** might support **different/unique** aspects of an overall goal for the same organization. The overall goal is presented as the center of the circle. In the filled-in example provided after the template the goal is to increase college readiness/access and enrollment and baccalaureate attainment for urban youth and returning adults. Using the various TRIO

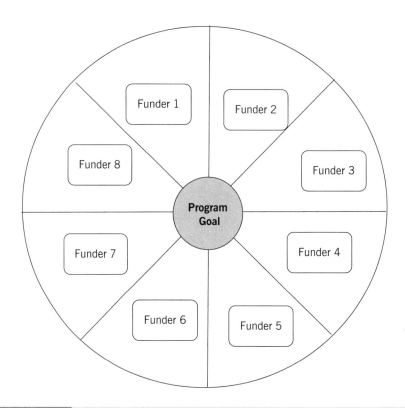

FIGURE 4.1a. Template for matching possible funders to program goals.

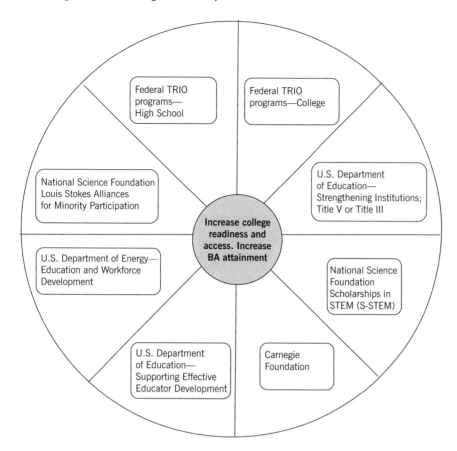

FIGURE 4.1b. Illustration for matching possible funders to program goals.

programs designed to serve low-income, first-generation students—including Talent Search, Upward Bound, and Student Support Services—the example demonstrates how one institution might have several funded programs at each level. In TRIO a single institution can submit multiple proposals under each competition as long as each proposal focuses on different schools/different populations.

Under the Talent Search regulations an institution of higher education may submit multiple applications as long as each project is serving students in different schools. The same is true for Upward Bound, and, in addition, multiple proposals can be submitted to serve different populations (regular, veterans, and disabled students). Finally, different student support services proposals can be submitted as long as each project serves a unique population (regular, teacher education, or science majors). As one aspect of this, a single institution can submit multiple Upward Bound proposals for funding as long as each grant is focused on a different population. So a college might submit a "regular" Upward Bound proposal, a "veterans" Upward Bound proposal, and an Upward Bound math and science proposal. It is theoretically possible that all three proposals could be funded because each serves a different population or different focus.

In similar fashion the Student Support Services RFP notes that a single institution may submit multiple proposals if each proposal serves a different focus group. Consequently, my college is able to have a "regular" Student Support Services project and a "Careers in Teaching" Student Support Services project.

CHAPTER SUMMARY

An essential step in developing a competitive proposal is to consider all of the aspects of the project you are considering by first expanding/broadening your conception of what you will want to accomplish, how you will accomplish it, and how you will know that you have succeeded. Once you have a broad view, you can begin to focus on the aspects that are realistically achievable, most critical to institutional success, appealing to funders, capacity building, and attainable. You want to perhaps consider a parsimonious approach and focus on activities that will yield the best outcomes for the largest population. Noted again in this chapter is the notion of "marketing" your project based on the preferences of the funder and how to choose the most appropriate/likely funder for your project. In some cases it is possible to submit multiple proposals to a funder if different populations are being served and to submit the same project to different funders for different aspects of a program approach. An example focuses on increasing college readiness, access, and completion for first-generation low-income students.

CHAPTER 5

Finding Funding

LEARNING OBJECTIVES

- How can I find funding for institutional/organizational priorities?
- What are the grant search websites and how can I use them?
- Do I have to sign up to use a grant submission website?
- How do I establish an account?
- What are the primary grant funding federal agencies and what do they support?

There are two ways to approach finding funding. If you have institutional priorities and needs that have been developed, you can use the grant search engines listed in this chapter to find possible RFPs that fit your priorities. Alternatively, you can find, through research or notifications, RFPs that are available with due dates in the near or far future and match your institutional or research needs to those opportunities.

Once you have chosen the programmatic, research, or project areas for proposal development and submission, the next step is to identify likely funding sources. There are a plethora of available databases and search engines through which funding opportunities can be located. For the vast majority the single and most convenient entry point is the Internet. This chapter presents information on the most commonly used sites and includes federal, foundation, and corporate sources. As each of the funders is likely to have its own unique requirements, a sampling is listed along with the types

Submitting Proposals

All proposals, with few exceptions, must be submitted electronically. If your organization has a legitimate case for submitting its proposal some other way, application to submit by mail or in person must be filed well in advance of the deadline so that it can be reviewed and a decision made before the due date. Specific instructions for requesting approval are provided in every RFP.

of projects funders seek to support, who is eligible, the URL to access their grant site, some information about the process of submission, and other information as warranted.

The federal government uses two web portals for grant submission, and each has unique aspects as well as a registration process that takes about 2 weeks to complete before you can sign on to use the site to submit a proposal. There are boxes within this chapter that review the process for G5 and Grants.gov as well as for several other unique sites. Also, Appendix B provides the URL for a website that explains how to use Grants.gov.

Using the Internet

The Internet is a necessary tool for finding and submitting grants. Few U.S. government departments or foundations accept paper submissions, and for most government grant competitions even nonfederal readers log on to review and score applications. The Internet can also be a source for ideas, strategies, and approaches for program design and evaluation. Finally, as we shall see in Chapter 10, the Internet is invaluable for finding the information required to support the need for funding in your community. Several sites useful for finding current competitions will be reviewed and explained. All of the information needed to use these resources is contained in this chapter.

If my institution or an organization we are partnering with is interested in a specific grant competition, the Internet is a valuable resource you can use to look at websites for funded projects. These project websites often provide information on their application forms, activities, outcome measures, and participants. The funder websites provided in the tables at the end of this chapter also post abstracts of funded programs over several years and are a resource for what activities are funded by the federal program.

There are a variety of Internet and subscription publications that may be helpful. Some are free for download from the Internet, but some are costly. An asterisk (*) in the paragraphs that follow indicates that there is a charge. In general, the costs are high but may be worthwhile if the resource is available for others at your institution. Many focus on specific areas such as education, health, social work, and business. They include:

● *Education Grants Alert* (Arlington, VA). Produced by LRP Publications, this is a weekly publication that lists grants available in education. LRP also sells books for grant seekers. These include *Get That Grant: Your Guide to Planning Successful K–12 Grant Proposals* by Gina Weisblat and *The Grants Glossary: An Educator's Guide to Codes, Terms and Tools* by Pam Moore. The website URL is **www.shoplrp.com. (*)**

● *Annual Register of Grant Support* (Medford, NJ). Information Today, Inc., is an annual directory now in its 41st edition. This publication is expensive, but it covers a wide range of areas. The website is **http://books.infotoday.com/ directories/anreg.shtml.** (*)

- *Assistance Listings* (Washington, DC). This website provides up-to-date information on grants as well as information and hints for proposal writing. The CFDA website is updated biweekly as new or updated program information is received from federal agencies. The website URL is **https://beta.sam. gov.**

- *Federal Register* (Washington, DC). The *Federal Register,* published on a daily basis by the Government Printing Office, contains government agency rules, proposed rules, and public notices. Its website allows the user to access this information. It is rather difficult to use but is a current and accurate source of information. The website URL is **www.federalregister.gov.**

- *Foundation Directory* (New York, NY). The Foundation Center offers online searching for foundation funding opportunities as well as online training and tutorials and tools and resources for grant seeking. These resources include specialized publications. Monthly subscriptions are available, and 3-month and yearly subscriptions offer cost savings. The website URL is **http://foundationcenter.org.** (*)

- *Forecast of Funding Opportunities.* Published by the U.S. Department of Education, this is a guide to potential programs anticipated to issue RFPs in the coming year. It is updated on a regular basis and is a good overview of what might be available. The website URL is **www2.ed.gov/fund/grant/find/ edlite-forecast.html.**

USING THE *FEDERAL REGISTER*

The *Federal Register* is the official daily publication for rules, proposed rules, and notices of federal agencies and organizations. It is published Monday through Friday, except federal holidays. *Federal Register* volumes from 59 (1994) to the present are available online.

Documents are available in Summary, PDF, ASCII text, or HTML format. HTML documents are available from 2000 forward and provide hypertext links to websites mentioned in the *Federal Register* document. Grant information is one of the most frequently searched-for materials from the *Federal Register*.

To use the *Federal Register,* go to **www. federalregister.gov**. This will take you to the main page, and you will be able to easily search on the current volume or on a range of volumes. You can also sign up to receive the daily Federal Register Table of Contents, but it is far easier to search on, for example, "education grants" or "first-generation college students," or "childhood obesity prevention grants." Once you obtain a list of possible documents, you can select to see the material in HTML, PDF, or in Summary form.

This is not the quickest, most effective, or efficient method to find grant funding opportunities, but it does offer some insight into the wide range of opportunities and documents published by the government every day of the week. As you will see in the descriptions of federal government departments and foundations, each department and foundation has information on the specific funding it offers, so looking at funding opportunities at the agency site is easier.

USING THE FORECAST OF FUNDING OPPORTUNITIES

The U.S. Department of Education, **www.ed.gov,** is comprised of a number of principal units, each of which oversees particular areas of grant funding. It issues the Forecast of Funding Opportunities at regular intervals to inform the public of the funding opportunities available for the foreseeable future as well as funding opportunities that have already closed. In most cases closed opportunities will likely be reopened with a similar deadline for the following year. This resource can be found at **www2.ed.gov/fund/grant/find/edlite-forecast.html.** The latest date of publication is always listed at the top of the document, as it is published during the late summer and updated regularly from November through July.

The Forecast of Funding Opportunities also provides the *Federal Register* volume and page number of the solicitation so that interested individuals can go to the website for the *Federal Register* and find the actual document. Additional information is also provided in the forecast, including the actual or estimated date for publication of the notice; a link to the notice; the deadline date for transmitting a completed application; and whether the completed application must be transmitted electronically through **www.grants.gov** or through **grants.gov**. Finally, the program contact person is listed by name with e-mail address, fax, and phone number.

- *Grants.gov.* This website is very useful and provides information about preparing grants in its "Grants Learning Center," a search engine for finding grants by keyword, and training videos to assist a novice user in navigating the Grants.gov site. This site requires registration through a guided process. Grants.gov requires the user to change his or her password on a regular basis and will send e-mails to remind you. The website is **www.grants.gov.**

- *Community of Science/Pivot.* Subscriptions to this comprehensive database are institutional. Users whose colleges or universities have purchased access can automatically log on from any computer on the network. Once you log on from your institutional computer, you can register a user ID and password that will permit access from any computer. Recently, the Community of Science (COS) has added user training through webinars that can be viewed as they are broadcast or accessed once they have been aired. The types of sponsors include foundations, governments, corporations, and public agencies. Grants cover all disciplines and many purposes. The records in the database share a common format and entries are updated daily. There is also a standardized keyword list so that if you find an entry that is appropriate you can use the keywords to find other similar opportunities. A valuable aspect of COS is that a user can save up to 40 different search criteria to run and can track updates for 200 individual records. The website URL is **http://pivot.cos.com. (*)**

- *The Foundation Center.* The Foundation Center has a searchable database of nearly 100,000 foundations, corporate donors, and grant-making public charities in the United States as well as listings of its most recent grants. Individuals can freely search the database but can access only limited information without an institutional or individual subscription. Interestingly subscriptions

BEFORE USING GRANTS.GOV

Before using Grants.gov, you or your organization must register, which requires a DUNS number. DUNS, the Data Universal Numbering System, is Dun & Bradstreet's proprietary system of identifying business entities on a location-specific basis. It is highly recommended that you complete this step with the assistance of the Office of Research and Sponsored Programs (Grants Office). The DUNS number is assigned by Dun & Bradstreet to businesses (including individuals doing business as sole proprietors). This number is permanent and remains with the company to which it has been assigned even if the company closes or goes out of business. It was adopted as the standard business identifier for federal electronic commerce (including grants and contracts) in 1994 and, in April 1998, as the federal government's contractor identification code for all procurement-related activities.

Once the DUNS number is assigned, which can take as long as 2 weeks, the organization or individual must register with the Central Contractor Registry (CCR) at **https://uscontractor-registration.com**. The CCR is the primary vendor database for the U.S. federal government. It collects, validates, stores, and disseminates data in support of agency acquisition missions. Both current and potential government vendors are required to register with the CCR in order to be awarded contracts/grants.

Finally, to submit a grant proposal as part of an organization there must be a person registered as an Authorized Organization Representative (AOR) through your organization. Once these steps are accomplished, you can register on Grants.gov. Until you complete them you cannot work on the site to prepare proposals and cannot submit proposals.

Note. In many cases there is a local grant management software program into which the principal investigator/proposal author uploads the required grant documents. The software also enables the routing of the proposal to various required signatories prior to final AOR approval and submission. If this is not the case, your organization will have to complete the registration process before you can log on to get the application materials and complete a grant submission. A completed application includes basic applicant information, required certifications and assurances, and a variety of separate forms and narrative content specified in the grant application. There are nine steps to submitting an application through Grants.gov, but the critical first steps for registration and authorization are essential. These are reviewed in **www.grants.gov/web/grants/learn-grants/grants-101.html**.

can be purchased on a monthly or yearly basis, enabling a subscriber to have short-term access to determine if the database is useful. The website URL is **http://foundationcenter.org**. (★)

• *Sponsored Program Information Network.* When I first began using a searchable grant database, this was the one my college used. At the time it was based at a university and was in development. It is now under the auspices of InfoEd, Inc. and is a full-service, fee-based site that offers electronic research administration including downloading application packages, proposal preparation, within-organization routing, and submission to the funding agency.

InfoEd's Sponsored Program Information Network (SPIN) contains information on grants, contracts, sabbatical opportunities, publication support, and curriculum development funding from over 6,000 entities. It also has several levels of query options from the most basic to the most advanced. As with COS,

USING THE FOUNDATION CENTER

The Foundation Center, located at **http://foundationcenter.org,** was established in 1956 and is today recognized as a leading authority on foundation funding. The Center has the most complete database on U.S. grant makers and provides many information resources as well as conducting free and affordable educational programs. It maintains an online subscription database that includes detailed information about U.S. foundations and corporate donors and grants.

The Foundation Center has library/learning centers in New York City; Washington, DC; Atlanta; Cleveland; and San Francisco that provide access to their extensive database and offer classes on funding research and writing.

Individuals, colleges, and community organizations can subscribe to its online database. The cost can be monthly or yearly. For example, a subscription that provides access to 10,000 foundations and 2 million grants costs $199.98/month, and you can cancel at any time. Current payment options can be found at **https://subscribe.foundationcenter.org/#/fdo/sign-up/professional.**

The Foundation Center offers a full spectrum of classroom and online classes as well as webinars that cover research on funding, proposal writing, and grant makers and giving, as well as publishing a wide variety of books on the funding process.

it permits users to set up an alert system that sends a notification about relevant programs that match their profile. Finally, the search engine is fully integrated with modules for proposal development, internal review, and submission.

The InfoEd system also permits the user to upload a curriculum vitae and academic profile. This information is searchable by others, and so can serve to enable you to find others in your areas of interest or enable others to find you. The website URL is **https://spin.infoedglobal.com.** (*)

• *American Federation of Teachers Listing of Grants and Awards.* This listing provides links to a number of opportunities pertinent to education. Each item enables the user to click through to a fuller explanation on the AFT website and then to the funder website. A review of opportunities may stimulate your thinking and enable you to broaden the scope of your project. The website URL is **www.aft.org.**

Individual Funding Agency Grant Databases

All government funding agencies have websites that feature grant opportunity deadlines and official RFPs. The sites also offer access to application packages and forms. In most cases previously funded projects are listed and sometimes summarized on the sites. This provides insight into the areas of funding, types of organizations funded, limitations on funding, and scope of funding. It also provides a breadth of ideas and topics in the areas the agency funds and enables the potential applicant to add additional ideas into the mix of information that is defining of the proposed project. Almost all funding agencies offer the opportunity for you to sign up to receive notifications of available funding and any modification or changes to current RFPs. These notifications can include new opportunities, RFPs in development, or changes in deadlines, priorities, and funding amounts. The sites also offer links to webinars or PowerPoints to help you understand the requirements of the proposals.

Corporate Foundation Websites

Corporate foundation grant opportunities are frequently embedded in the overall corporate website, and a quick search of their site using "grants" as the keyword will provide a link to the information you need. All of the information needed to apply, including the application form, is on the website and includes areas of interest; grant guidelines; due dates; available funding; and previously funded project abstracts. Often corporate foundations indicate that "unsolicited applications are not accepted." If this is the case, they may accept letters of inquiry that are reviewed and if found appropriate can lead to a solicitation for an application.

Federal Funding Agencies

United States government agencies offer funding opportunities for programs within their purview. Many of them are listed below. Each agency issues its own RFPs with varying submission guidelines and regulations. The materials at the end of this chapter include a table for each agency featuring information pertinent to federal funding using a template that assures consistent organization of material. There are, as we have seen, several approaches to finding project/program funding. Each approach/method has strengths and weaknesses. This chapter presents an overview of government funding agencies and describes each of the major funding sources; provides the URL to access the department/agency; and briefly describes the types of funding opportunities, who is eligible to apply, the process of applying, and other pertinent information as needed. The chart on page 52 shows the federal agencies included, the table number, and the page.

Grant opportunities from the federal government are announced daily Monday through Friday in the *Federal Register,* which can be accessed at **www.federalregister.gov.**

However, this is a cumbersome approach, as the *Federal Register* is a record of all speeches, resolutions, actions, and announcements. Fortunately, there is a method of searching that can speed your access to areas of interest. This search capability is found at **www.federalregister.gov** and at **www.grants.gov.**

Both of these approaches are problematic and it is far better to go directly to a government department that is likely to fund projects/programs in your area of interest. Each of the government agencies that is of interest to grant developers and writers is described below, and pertinent information on their funding opportunities is presented in individual tables.

Summary of Tables for Federal Funding Agencies

Agency	Table No.	Page No.
Agency for International Development (USAID)	5.1	58
Corporation for National and Community Service (CNCS)	5.2	59
Department of Agriculture (USDA)	5.3	60
Department of Commerce (DOC)	5.4	61
Department of Defense (DOD)	5.5	62
Department of Education (USDE)	5.6	63
Department of Health and Human Services (HHS)	5.7	64
Department of Housing and Urban Development (HUD)	5.8	65
Department of Justice (DOJ)	5.9	66
Department of Labor (DOL)	5.10	67
Department of State (DOS)	5.11	68
Environmental Protection Agency (EPA)	5.12	69
National Aeronautics and Space Agency (NASA)	5.13	70
National Endowment for the Arts (NEA)	5.14	71
National Endowment for the Humanities (NEH)	5.15	72
National Institutes of Health (NIH)	5.16	73
National Science Foundation (NSF).	5.17	74

Agency for International Development

The USAID believes that we live in an era that has seen dramatic change in recent years—an era that is rapidly evolving. Globalization, technology, HIV/AIDS, rapid population growth, terrorism, conflict, weapons of mass destruction, and failing states—these are just some of the issues shaping today's world. Most of these issues—both good and bad—do not recognize national borders. They affect us directly and are dramatically altering the way in which we think and operate.

Corporation for National and Community Service

The CNCS plays a vital role in supporting the American culture of citizenship, service, and responsibility. The CNCS is a catalyst for change and champion for the ideal that every American has skills and talents to give. It is the nation's largest grant maker supporting service and volunteering. Through its Senior Corps, AmeriCorps, and Learn and Serve America programs, it provides opportunities for Americans of all ages and backgrounds to express their patriotism while addressing critical community needs.

Department of Agriculture

Established in 1862, the USDA serves all Americans through anti-hunger efforts, stewardship of nearly 200 million acres of national forest and range-lands, and through product safety and conservation efforts. The USDA opens markets for American farmers and ranchers and provides food for needy people around the world.

Department of Commerce

The DOC fosters and promotes the nation's economic development and technological advancement through vigilance in international trade policy and domestic business policy and growth, and by promoting economic progress at all levels.

Department of Defense

The DOD provides the military forces needed to deter war and protect the security of the United States in five major areas: peacekeeping and war-fighting efforts, homeland security, evacuation planning, and humanitarian causes.

Department of Education

The USDE ensures equal access to education and promotes educational excellence through coordination, management, and accountability in federal education programs. The department works to supplement and complement educational efforts on all levels, encouraging increased involvement by the public, parents, and students.

Department of Health and Human Services

HHS is the federal government's principal agency for protecting the health of all Americans and providing essential human services, especially to those who are least able to help themselves.

Department of Housing and Urban Development

HUD's mission is to create strong, sustainable, inclusive communities and quality affordable homes for all. HUD is working to strengthen the housing market to bolster the economy and protect consumers; meet the need for quality affordable rental homes; utilize housing as a platform for improving quality of life; build inclusive and sustainable communities free from discrimination; and transform the way it does business.

Department of Justice

The DOJ offers funding opportunities to conduct research, support law enforcement activities in state and local jurisdictions, provide training and technical assistance, and implement programs that improve the criminal justice system. Discretionary grant funds are announced in the *Federal Register* or through program solicitations that can also be found through bureau and Office of Justice (OJP) websites. Funding Opportunities at OJP provides links to application kits, current funding opportunities listed by source, and the Grants Management System (GMS). Of particular use to new applicants, the OJP Grants 101 portal presents a step-by-step guide through the grant application process.

Department of Labor

The DOL fosters and promotes the welfare of job seekers, wage earners, and retirees by improving their working conditions, advancing their opportunities, protecting their retirement and health benefits, and generally protecting worker rights and monitoring national economic measures.

Department of State

The DOS strives to create a more secure, democratic, and prosperous world for the benefit of the American people and the international community.

Environmental Protection Agency

The mission of the EPA is to protect human health and the environment. Its purpose is to ensure that Americans are protected from significant risks to human health and the environment; efforts to reduce environmental risk are based on the best available scientific information; federal laws related to health and the environment are enforced; environmental protection is integral to U.S. policies; and all have access to accurate information on managing human health and environmental risks.

National Aeronautics and Space Agency

Supporting research in science and technology is an important part of NASA's overall mission. NASA solicits this research through the release of various research announcements in a wide range of science and technology disciplines. NASA uses a peer review process to evaluate and select research proposals submitted in response to these research announcements. Researchers can help

NASA achieve national research objectives by submitting research proposals and conducting awarded research. This site facilitates the search for NASA research opportunities.

National Endowment for the Arts

The NEA is a public agency dedicated to supporting excellence in the arts, bringing the arts to all Americans and providing leadership in arts education. The Endowment is the largest national source of funds for the arts.

National Endowment for the Humanities

The NEH typically funds projects at museums, archives, libraries, colleges, universities, public television, and radio stations, and for individual scholars. The grants are focused on strengthening teaching and learning, facilitating research and original scholarship; developing opportunities for lifelong learning; preserving and providing access to cultural and educational resources; and strengthening the humanities.

National Institutes of Health

The NIH, a part of the U.S. Department of Health and Human Services, is the primary federal agency for conducting and supporting medical research. Helping to lead the way toward important medical discoveries that improve people's health and save lives, NIH scientists investigate ways to prevent disease as well as the causes, treatments, and even cures for common and rare diseases. Composed of 27 institutes and centers, the NIH provides leadership and financial support to researchers in every state and throughout the world.

National Science Foundation

The NSF is the only federal agency that supports all fields of fundamental science and engineering. In addition to supporting traditional science research to keep the United States at the leading edge of discovery, the NSF also supports what it terms "high-risk, high pay-off" ideas and projects that may seem like science fiction today but may be the norm tomorrow. Their funding integrates research and education so that tomorrow's top scientists and researchers are prepared.

Corporate and Private Funders

Foundations take many forms: private, family, corporate, independent, public and community. Each has different rules, but all provide funding according to the interests and causes subscribed to by establishing parties. In applying to foundations for funding, it is usual that the grant seeker prepare a letter of inquiry appealing for support and highlighting how his or her project relates to the interests/causes of the foundation.

In addition, the applicant should provide a one-page overview of the project to be supported. Appendix B includes a link to a website that offers suggestions on how to approach foundations. Tables 5.18–5.33 provide information on foundations, including website, overview, ways to obtain funding, eligibility, types of funding, application process, and, if appropriate, additional helpful information. Many funders publish useful information, which will also be noted. The funders to be reviewed appear in the chart below.

There are many more foundations that can be found through the Foundation Center, on the Internet, and through various publications and e-mail updates. Some foundations, however, do not accept letters of inquiry or other solicitations for funding but rather prefer to focus grant making on continuing commitments in areas of focus.

Summary of Tables for Foundation Funding

Foundation name	Table no.	Page no.
Annie E. Casey Foundation	5.18	75
Carnegie Corporation of New York	5.19	76
Charles Stewart Mott Foundation	5.20	77
ExxonMobil Foundation	5.21	78
Ford Foundation	5.22	79
Gates Foundation	5.23	80
IBM Community Foundation	5.24	81
J. P. Morgan Chase	5.25	82
Metropolitan Life Foundation	5.26	83
Pew Charitable Trust	5.27	84
Robert Wood Johnson Foundation	5.28	85
Alfred P. Sloan Foundation	5.29	86
Rockefeller Foundation	5.30	87
Spencer Foundation	5.31	88
Verizon Foundation	5.32	89
W. K. Kellogg Foundation	5.33	90

Therefore they do not review unsolicited letters of inquiry or proposals. So in searching for foundation funding the grant seeker needs to read all information carefully to determine what areas of interest for funding are listed, whether funding is limited to ongoing projects, whether letters of inquiry are required, and whether they should be sent online or by mail and if any letters of inquiry or unsolicited proposals are accepted.

CHAPTER SUMMARY

This chapter identifies several approaches to searching for RFPs and includes instructions for how to use Internet sites that provide funding information. Some Internet sites require a subscription (and are quite expensive), but many useful sites are free. Government funders (both state and federal) have websites that detail opportunities, policies, priorities, and programs. Information on 17 government funding agencies is presented, including website, overview, how to find funding, eligibility, types of funding, application process, and other information. The same types of information are given for 16 foundations.

TABLE 5.1. Agency for International Development (USAID)

Website	www.usaid.gov
Overview	The USAID works in agriculture, democracy and governance, economic growth, the environment, education, and health, and supports global partnerships and humanitarian assistance in more than 100 countries to provide a better future for all. Colleges and universities or public schools that partner with agencies in host countries can develop grant proposals to fund their collaborative work.
Finding funding	As with other government agencies all submissions to USAID must be through Grants.gov. The USAID website provides background and insight on opportunities, though funding opportunities can be found at Grants.gov as well. The website also provides specific information for grant and partnership programs at **www.usaid.gov/work-usaid/partnership-opportunities/search-for-opportunities**.
Who is eligible	Colleges, universities, and other partners that work with agencies in host countries. The application must come from the host country in partnership with an eligible entity.
Types of funding	Health, education, agriculture, infrastructure development, program planning, environment, global hunger and food security, economic opportunity, social and economic services for vulnerable populations, and program design and learning.
Process	The agency also provides assistance in the design, award, and administration of results-oriented grants and cooperative agreements to implement foreign assistance activities. This information is designed as a "user-friendly" resource for USAID staff and development partners (e.g., private voluntary organizations [PVOs], nongovernmental organizations [NGOs], cooperative development organizations, educational institutions, and private firms) on USAID's programming policies and procedures. It can be accessed at **www.usaid.gov/work-usaid/how-to-work-with-usaid**.
Other information	The USAID website includes a web page that provides information on how to work with USAID. It is recommended reading for all considering applying for funding. This can be accessed at **www.usaid.gov/work-usaid/how-to-work-with-usaid**.

TABLE 5.2. Corporation for National and Community Service (CNCS)

Website	www.nationalservice.gov
Overview	The programs of this agency support service and volunteering through Senior Corps, AmeriCorps, and Learn and Serve America programs with grants to K–12 School-Based Programs; Higher Education Programs; Innovative and Community-Based Service-Learning Programs; and Programs for Native American Communities. The agency is a catalyst for change and offers every American a chance to contribute through service and volunteering.
Finding funding	Grants available through the Corporation for National and Community Service are described on the website by type of funding. However, applications for programs must be completed at **www.g5.gov.** In order to use this site you must be registered.
Who is eligible	Elementary K–3; Elementary 4–6; Middle School 6–8; High School 9–12; Higher Education; Community-Based Organizations; Tribes/U.S. Territories. Learn and Serve America provides direct and indirect support to K–12 schools, community groups, and higher education institutions to facilitate service-learning projects. Projects that combine classroom curriculum with community service are of particular interest.
Types of funding	Program areas are organized as follows: K–12 School-Based Programs, Higher Education Programs, Innovative and Community-Based Service-Learning Programs, Programs for Native American Communities, and Service-Learning Impact Study. Each of these areas has specific guidelines and opportunities. For example, K–12 school-based programs engage students in service-learning programs that aid young people (5–17), including those with disabilities, in applying academic content knowledge to meet critical community needs. Higher education programs support innovative service-learning programs carried out through higher education institutions to meet the human, educational, environmental, or public safety needs of neighboring communities. Similarly community-based organizations and Native American communities qualify for funding to develop and implement service learning projects.
Process	Locate the funding opportunity you want to respond to on the website and check the due date. Once the application is issued (released) it will be available for access at **www.g5.gov.**
Other information	The website has information designed to assist new and novice grant writers to prepare proposals. It also offers many resources at **www.nationalservice.gov/ build-your-capacity.** Many examples, research on outcomes of service learning, suggestions for projects, and a toolkit for organizing projects and finding funding make this a very user-friendly site.

TABLE 5.3. Department of Agriculture (USDA)

Website	**www.usda.gov** and **www.nifa.usda.gov/grants.**
Overview	One of the primary sections within the Department of Agriculture that funds projects and programs is the National Institute of Food and Agriculture (NIFA). The funding opportunities offered range from agricultural and food biosecurity through environmental and natural resources to technology and engineering. These areas of emphasis are listed on the search page to facilitate identification of appropriate opportunities. Another search criterion is program group, with four areas ranging from education to small business. The final criterion is eligibility group, which includes, among others, governments, IHE type, 501(c)(3) type.
Finding funding	The USDA/NIFA has a search site that can be used to find targeted grant opportunities. This is at **www.usda.gov/topics/research-and-science.**
Who is eligible	A wide variety of agencies, institutions, governments, and 501(c)(3)'s are eligible for various categories of funding. The search engine provided on the NIFA sites enables you to quickly find targeted opportunities.
Types of funding	The agency funds research projects on all aspects of food production, protection, safety, delivery, and consumption, community food, education and health related to food and nutrition, food science, pest management, crop management, and farming.
Process	All USDA grants are submitted through grants.gov. The process of applying for USDA funding, including information, e-mail update subscription, application checklist, sample application, and application guide, is provided at **www.usda. gov/topics/research-and-science**.
Other information	A guide to the USDA and a sample application can be found at **www.nifa.usda. gov/funding/sample.html**.

TABLE 5.4. Department of Commerce (DOC)

Website	www.commerce.gov
Overview	The Department of Commerce is comprised of several bureaus, including Bureau of Economic Analysis (BEA); Bureau of Industry and Security (BIS); U.S. Census Bureau; Economic Development Administration (EDA); Economics and Statistics Administration (ESA); International Trade Administration (ITA); Minority Business Development Agency (MBDA); National Oceanic and Atmospheric Administration (NOAA); National Telecommunications and Information Administration (NTIA); National Institute of Standards and Technology (NIST); National Technical Information Service (NTIS); and U.S. Patent and Trademark Office (USPTO).
Finding funding	The Department of Commerce funding opportunities are listed at Grants.gov. You can view solicitations if you search by agency and select Department of Commerce. Opportunities can also be viewed at **www.commerce.gov** by clicking on each of the Commerce Bureaus that offer grants and funding opportunities. These are EDA, NOAA, NTIA, and NIST. Each of the bureaus posts opportunities that are available.
Who is eligible	U.S. companies, academia, and other organizations conduct joint research and development projects are eligible to participate in Cooperative Research and Development Agreements. Each of the four bureaus that offer funding and/or cooperative partnerships present detailed information on eligibility within each opportunity.
Types of funding	There are several types of funding: grants for research and demonstration programs; guest researcher at a research laboratory; contracts for specific work; availability of laboratory facilities for specialized research.
Process	Applicants should use Grants.gov to download funding opportunities and to submit their proposal.
Other information	Several of the commerce bureaus have statistical profiles and reports that can be used to establish need and to describe communities and neighborhoods that might require funding-related projects.

TABLE 5.5. Department of Defense (DOD)

Website	**www.darpa.mil**
Overview	The section of the Department of Defense that oversees funding and contracts is the Defense Advanced Research Projects Agency (DARPA). To apply for funding, review DARPA's research interests, find suitable solicitations, and follow the instructions therein to submit your proposal. All of DARPA's research is performed by outside researchers at businesses (with some opportunities reserved for small businesses), universities, nonprofit institutions, government laboratories, and other research organizations.
Finding funding	DARPA announces its research needs through solicitations that most often take the form of a Broad Agency Announcement (BAA) but may also be called Special Notices, Research Announcements, or Requests for Proposals. Solicitations may be office specific or may involve multiple offices. Most opportunities are listed through Grants.gov.
Who is eligible	Businesses (with some opportunities reserved for small businesses), universities, nonprofit institutions, government laboratories, and other research organizations are eligible for funding. Some opportunities are restricted to certain organizations and this is clearly specified.
Types of funding	Areas of funding tend to be specific to technical offices. Opportunities encompass defense sciences, neuroergonomics, visual intelligence in machines, engineering, behavioral issues, robotics, strategic technology, tactical technology, basic, applied, and advanced space-related research projects, and information processing.
Process	The Defense Sciences Office welcomes new technical ideas at any time from all public and private entities and is currently soliciting proposals for advanced research and development in a variety of enabling technical areas. The DOD/DSO/DARPA Opportunities page provides information about current open solicitations, (**www.darpa.mil/work-with-us/opportunities**) to peruse emerging research interests. Before submitting a white paper or proposal, the DOD encourages you to discuss your idea with a DSO Program Manager. You can find the program manager by downloading the specific solicitation you are interested in pursuing.

TABLE 5.6. Department of Education (USDE)

Website	**www.ed.gov, www.grants.gov, www.g5.gov**
Overview	The Department of Education was created in 1980 by combining offices from several federal agencies. Its mission is to promote student achievement and preparation for global competitiveness by fostering educational excellence and ensuring equal access by establishing policies on federal financial aid for education, and distributing as well as monitoring those funds; collecting data on America's schools and disseminating research; focusing national attention on key educational issues; and prohibiting discrimination and ensuring equal access to education.
Finding funding	The Education Department administers its funding through **www.g5.gov,** and information on funding opportunities can be found there as well as through the department's website **www.ed.gov** and through **www.grants.gov.** The types of funding are (1) grants to help students attend college (students can use the Free Application for Federal Student Aid to apply for Pell Grants and other aid for college); (2) formula grants to agencies using formulas determined by Congress, which have no application process; and (3) discretionary grants to organizations, agencies, and individuals (these are awarded using a competitive process—anyone who meets the eligibility requirements can apply). Funding opportunities can also be found through the following sources: Guide to Education Programs: Discretionary Grant Application Packages; the *Federal Register*; the Forecast of Funding Opportunities; and Grants.gov.
Who is eligible	Eligibility for funding is clearly stated within each of the Requests for Proposals. However, for most of the grant opportunities eligible institutions include schools, school districts, states, institutions of higher education, charter schools, local education agencies, nonprofits with or without 501(c)(3) status, Hispanic Serving Institutions, Minority Serving Institutions, Historically Black Colleges and Universities, and Native American tribal governments. For a quick look at eligibility you can go to Grants.gov, search by agency, click on a particular competition, and scroll down to eligible applicants.
Types of funding	The sections within the Forecast of Funding Opportunities define the range of areas and types of funding available. **www2.ed.gov/fund/grant/find/edlite-forecast.html** The individual charts in the forecast cover: Chart 1—Institute of Education Sciences. Chart 2—Office of Elementary and Secondary Education. Chart 3—Office of Innovation and Improvement. Chart 4—Office of Postsecondary Education (Link to IFLE Chart) Chart 5—Office of Special Education and Rehabilitative Services (Links to RSA Chart) Chart 6—Office of Career, Technical and Adult Education Chart 7—Office of English Language Acquisition
Process	A potential applicant for funding must register at **www.g5.gov** well in advance of the application due date since all inquiries and application packages are accessed through the website and proposals and related documentation must be submitted through the website as well.
Other information	The Department of Education published a strategic plan outlining its goals for 2018–2022. It is an interesting document and highlights many of the objectives that are critical for many of the funding opportunities. It can be accessed at **www2.ed.gov/about/reports/strat/index.html.** The website also provides access to initiatives of the current president and administration and is useful in preparing proposals that address their priorities. Also included and of interest are the administration's high-priority performance goals.

TABLE 5.7. Department of Health and Human Services (HHS)

Website	www.hhs.gov
Overview	The department's programs are administered by 11 operating divisions, including eight agencies in the U.S. Public Health Service and three human services agencies. The department operates more than 300 programs, covering a wide spectrum of activities. In addition to the services they deliver, the HHS programs provide for equitable treatment of beneficiaries nationwide, and they enable the collection of national health and other data.
Finding funding	Links on the DHHS site enable the user to find available HHS grant opportunities (Grants.gov); search/browse forecasted HHS grant opportunities (GrantsForecast); or find funding opportunities for faith-based and community organizations (FBCI). Alternatively the user can go to Grants.gov and search by funding agency.
Who is eligible	Communities, educational institutions, states, cities, local agencies, hospitals, Indian reservations, health departments, and libraries.
Types of funding	DHHS provides funding opportunities in a wide variety of areas including community development; education; employment, labor, and training; environmental quality research and education; health; and income security and social services. There are a total of 700+ grant opportunities listed across the categories.
Process	See the general process for submitting grants through Grants.gov.
Other information	The DHHS has several links on its website to help individuals write and manage HHS grants. These include tips for preparing proposals, grant management procedures, and general information about the HHS grants management process. The site also enables users to see grants by major activity type, operating division, and recipient class.

TABLE 5.8. Department of Housing and Urban Development (HUD)

Website	**www.hud.gov**
Overview	The Department of Housing and Urban Development's mission is to sustain homeownership, support community development, and increase access to affordable housing free from discrimination. Grant opportunities contribute to this mission through a series of cross-cutting priorities that include job creation, sustainability, fair housing, capacity building/knowledge sharing, and using housing to improve other outcomes and expand cross-cutting policy knowledge.
Finding funding	As is the case with many government grants, HUD applications go through Grants.gov, but information can be found at the department site: **www.hud. gov/grants.** There you will find information about and links to the available competitions.
Who is eligible	Higher education institutions classified as HBCUs, HSIs, tribal colleges, and Alaska Native and Native Hawaiian institutions, as well as communities, through community and economic development programs, affordable housing, and special needs assistance.
Types of funding	Programs fund higher education institutions working with communities and target HBCUs, Hispanic-Serving Institutions Assisting Communities (HSIACs), Alaska Native/Native Hawaiian Institutions Assisting Communities (AN/NHIAC), tribal colleges and universities, and doctoral dissertation research grant programs. HUD also has an Office of University Partnerships, which provides information, publications, and features on funding. The URL is **www.hud.gov/program_ offices/spm/gmomgmt/grantsinfo.** There is also funding for community development work–study programs, community outreach partnership centers, and Universities Rebuilding America partnerships. Community funding includes YouthBuild, community block grants, empowerment zones, and economic development loan guarantees.
Process	HUD grants are applied for through Grants.gov. The Grants.gov process is described in detail in Chapter 5. In addition, several videos have been prepared for novice users. A webinar prepared in 2017 is also helpful (**www.youtube.com/ watch?v=0G3LPykslCg&t=240s**).
Other information	In conjunction with HUD you can use American Factfinder to obtain information about programs, needs, population, and housing, and state, federal, and local statistics (**https://factfinder.census.gov**). In addition, HUD has links to its grants office, competitive funding opportunities, funding announcements (so you can see what types of projects were funded), and highest-scoring applications (to illustrate firsthand what they are seeking). Their site also has links to training webcasts related to grants.

TABLE 5.9. Department of Justice (DOJ)

Website	**www.justice.gov**
Overview	The Office of Justice Programs offers federal financial assistance to scholars, practitioners, experts, and state and local governments and agencies as well as formula grants to state agencies that subgrant funds to units of state and local government. Discretionary grant funds are announced in the *Federal Register* or through program solicitations that can also be found through the bureau and OJP websites. The website at **https://ojp.gov/funding** provides links to application kits, current funding opportunities listed by source, and the Grants Management System (GMS).
Finding funding	A very useful feature of the OJP website is the step-by-step guide through the grant application process called Grants 101 found at **www.ojp.gov/grants101.** Of special interest for grant seekers are the opportunities available through congressionally directed awards and discretionary grants. Although grant applications must be made through **www.grants.gov,** the OJP has 10 areas of interest under which related funding can be found. These are summarized below but are also at **www.grantsnet.justice.gov/programplan/html/Home.htm.**
Who is eligible	Eligibility depends upon the particular competition: Bureau of Justice Assistance, Office of Juvenile Justice and Delinquency Prevention. Eligibility requirements are summarized in each program area.
Types of funding	The areas under which OJP funding is organized are detailed under its program plan and include the following areas: preventing crime and empowering communities to address crime; breaking the cycles of mental illness, substance abuse, and crime; preventing and intervening in juvenile offending and victimization; managing offenders to reduce recidivism and promote successful reentry; effective interventions to address violence, victimization, and victims' rights; enhancing law enforcement initiatives; supporting innovation in adjudication; countering terrorism and addressing domestic emergencies; advancing technology to prevent and solve crime; and innovations in justice information sharing.
Process	The process of applying for a grant from OJP is also detailed on the site and can be accessed at **https://ojp.gov/funding/Apply/GrantProcess.htm**
Other information	Agencies within the DOJ, listed below, also have sites that provide grant information specific to each agency. Programs, funding opportunities, application assistance, and other useful information can be found on these sites. Bureau of Justice Assistance (BJA) Bureau of Justice Statistics (BJS) Community Capacity Development Office (CCDO) National Criminal Justice Reference Service (NCJRS) National Institute of Justice (NIJ) Office of Juvenile Justice and Delinquency Prevention (OJJDP) Office of Sex Offender Sentencing, Monitoring, Apprehending, Registering, and Tracking (SMART) Office for Victims of Crime (OVC)

TABLE 5.10. Department of Labor (DOL)

Website	**www.dol.gov**
Overview	The department of labor is comprised of several sections, including the Occupational Safety and Health Administration (OSHA)
Finding funding	Department of Labor funding opportunities can be found through its website or through Grants.gov by clicking on "find grant opportunities," browsing by agency, and choosing Department of Labor. Generally the DOL has limited funding opportunities, as much of its funds are allocated through states.
Who is eligible	The types of organizations that are eligible to receive grants include nonprofit and community/faith-based organizations, employer associations, labor unions, joint labor/management associations, and colleges and universities.
Types of funding	Training and education programs aimed at identifying workplace hazards, understanding worker rights and responsibilities, protecting health and saving lives through safety and health training, and educational programs for workers and employers.
Process	As with many other U.S. government funding opportunities, the process entails registering with Grants.gov or using the institutional registration. The application package must be downloaded through the Grants.gov website and submitted in advance of the deadline day and time to be considered. Guidelines for electronic grant submission can be accessed at **www.grants.gov/web/grants/learn-grants/grants-101.html.**

TABLE 5.11. Department of State (DOS)

Website	www.state.gov
Overview	The mission of the Grants Division (ECA-IIP/EX/G) is to effectively plan, direct, and execute by grant or cooperative agreement, or other appropriate means, assistance instruments for the department's educational and cultural exchange programs. The department's agreements support academic, cultural, and professional exchange and training programs as a means of seeking mutual understanding between the people of the United States and the people of other countries and promoting the free exchange of information and ideas.
Finding funding	Department of State funding opportunities can be found through its website.
Who is eligible	Eligibility varies according to type of grant but generally includes public and state-controlled institutions of higher education, not-for-profits with or without 501(c)(3) status, private institutions of higher education, for-profit organizations other than small businesses, and small businesses.
Types of funding	Many of the grant solicitations of the Department of State are found under the Bureau of Educational and Cultural Affairs and are largely comprised of exchange programs. The Department of State also oversees the Fulbright exchange programs, the *Hubert H. Humphrey Fellowship Program,* community college initiatives, and the *Benjamin A. Gilman International Scholarship Program* with the assistance of private, nonprofit organizations. Also administered within the Department of State are a wide range of grants in other areas including English Language Teaching and Learning, the International Visitor Leadership Program, the Summer Work/Travel Program, Professional Exchanges, Youth Programs, Sports United, and cultural programs.
Process	The Department of State includes helpful documents on its website at **http://exchanges.state.gov/pro-admin.html** with advice on funding opportunities. These documents include *The Bureau of Educational and Cultural Affairs Grant Process* (PDF); *Proposal Solicitation Eligibility and Process* (PDF); *Making Your Grant Proposal Competitive* (PDF); and *Grantee Recipients—Alumni Outreach, Tracking and Engagement* (PDF). Generally, however, acquisition of Requests for Grant Proposals (RFGPs) is best done through Grants.gov, where applications may be downloaded and printed and where grant proposals and the required parts and pieces must be uploaded by the specified date and time deadline.

TABLE 5.12. Environmental Protection Agency

Website	www.epa.gov
Overview	The mission of the EPA is to protect human health and the environment by ensuring that all Americans are protected from significant risks to human health and the environment where they live, learn, and work; environmental risk is scientifically studied and reduced; laws pertinent to the mission of EPA are enforced; environmental protection is considered as an integral part of U.S. policies; universal access to accurate information is provided; and communities and ecosystems are diverse, sustainable, and economically productive.
Finding funding	Research and funding efforts for the EPA are guided by the National Center for Environmental Research at **www.epa.gov/ncer** and can be located by clicking through to grants and funding. As in previous cases grant opportunities can also be located at grants.gov through searching by agency.
Who is eligible	Eligibility varies for different competitions but generally academic and nonprofit institutions located in the United States, and state and local governments are included.
Types of funding	Funding is available for Science to Achieve Results (STAR) Research Grants, EPA and other National Center for Environmental Research competitions; and EPA Environmental Research Fellowships. Further categories of funding include Biodiversity, Collaborative Science and Technology for Sustainability, Experimental Programs to Stimulate Competitive Research, Environmental Technology, and People, Prosperity, and the Planet—a student design competition for sustainability.
Process	The website at **www.epa.gov/ncer/rfa/forms/index.html** provides all forms needed to apply for various type of grants/funding.
Other information	The EPA site also provides a list of science topics of interest to encourage individuals to submit proposals in areas of national need. These include Community Risk Assessment; Children's Centers; Drinking Water; Ecological Science; Endocrine Disruptors; Global Change; and Technology for a Sustainable Environment.

TABLE 5.13. National Aeronautics and Space Agency (NASA)

Website	www.nasa.gov and http://nspires.nasaprs.com/external
Overview	NASA's mission is to pioneer the future in space exploration, scientific discovery, and aeronautics research. Throughout its history NASA has conducted or funded research that has improved life on earth. NASA funds both research and education. The research leads to discoveries and solutions; the education is focused on preparing new generations of students for careers in STEM fields related to aeronautics and space exploration.
Finding funding	NASA organizes its projects for educators according to grade level: K–4, 5–8, 9–12, higher education, and informal education. At the website various programs under each category are listed.
Who is eligible	Eligible applicants include institutions of higher education, other nonprofits, K–12 public and independent schools and school systems, and state, local, and Indian tribal governments in the United States.
Types of funding	NASA's Office of Education, in collaboration with the Mission Directorates, issues NRAs that solicit projects that (1) foster formal education goals (e.g., attract and retain students in STEM disciplines); (2) engage self-directed learners in NASA's mission; and/or (3) contribute to participation by minority organizations, small businesses, and disadvantaged small businesses across NASA's full portfolio of education programs (i.e., e-education, elementary and secondary education, higher education, and informal education).
Process	Applications for NASA programs must be submitted through **http://grants.gov.** Initially all available funding announcements can be accessed through the NASA website according to the grade level of interest or by informal science institutions. The full announcement can be obtained from the website as well as all materials related to the grant application. Submissions must be made through the Grants.gov site by the due date and time of the grant.
Other information	A guidebook for proposers titled *Responding to a NASA Research Announcement (NRA) or Cooperative Agreement Notice (CAN)* is available at **www.hq.nasa.gov/office/procurement/nraguidebook.**

TABLE 5.14. National Endowment for the Arts (ARTS)

Website	www.arts.gov
Overview	The National Endowment for the Arts is a public agency dedicated to supporting excellence in the arts, both new and established; bringing the arts to all Americans; and providing leadership in arts education. Established by Congress in 1965 as an independent agency of the federal government, the Endowment is the nation's largest annual funder of the arts, encouraging creativity through support of performances, exhibitions, festivals, artist residencies, and other arts projects throughout the country.
Finding funding	The NEA site for finding grant opportunities, at **https://www.arts.gov/grants** is organized according to disciplines in the arts. The areas included are artist communities, arts education, dance, design, folk and traditional arts, literature, local arts agencies, media arts, museums, music, musical theater, opera, presentations, state and regional theater, and the visual arts. Within each area there are several grant opportunities described with links to specific restrictions, guidelines, and expected outcomes. Also helpful are links to what an applicant needs to know: **www.arts.gov/grants/apply-grant/grants-organizations.**
Who is eligible	Almost all NEA grant funding goes to institutions and organizations. Under federal law, only a few categories of NEA funding are available for direct grants to individuals. These fund Literature Fellowships, NEA Jazz Masters Fellowships, NEA National Heritage Fellowships in the Folk and Traditional Arts, and National Endowment for the Arts Opera Honors.
Types of funding	There are a broad range of opportunities within each of the funding areas listed above. As an example, for arts education, the following opportunities are listed: Learning in the Arts for Children and Youth; Access to Artistic Excellence; Challenge America Fast-Track Review Grants; Creativity and Aging in America: Lifelong Learning in the Arts; the Arts on Radio and Television; the NEA Mayor's Institute on City Design 25th Anniversary Initiative; Coming Up Taller; and the National Endowment for the Arts Education Leaders Institute.
Process	The NEA accepts funding applications through Grants.gov. The process of using Grants.gov can be accessed at **www.grants.gov/web/grants/learn-grants/grants-101.html.** Briefly, you must register for Grants.gov and can then log on to search for new funding opportunities. The announcement has the date on which the application is available as well as the date on which your proposal must be in the system to qualify for review.
Other information	The NEA also publishes helpful articles that are intended to assist potential grantees to submit fundable proposals. These can be found at: **www.arts.gov/publications.** In addition a link is provided to an extensive database of awards, services, and publications for artists in all disciplines at the New York Foundation for the Arts. The link is **www.arts.gov/grants/recent-grants.**

TABLE 5.15. National Endowment for the Humanities (NEH)

Website	www.neh.gov
Overview	The National Endowment for the Humanities serves and strengthens our country by promoting excellence in the humanities and conveying the lessons of history to all Americans. The Endowment accomplishes this mission by providing grants for high-quality humanities projects in four funding areas: preserving and providing access to cultural resources, education, research, and public programs.
Finding funding	The NEH listing of funding opportunities is organized by area under the following headings: "Bridging Cultures"; "Challenge Grants"; "Education Programs"; "Federal/State Partnerships"; "Office of Digital Humanities"; "Preservation and Access"; "Public Programs"; "Research Programs"; and "We the People." Under each area specific opportunities are listed. For education programs, for example, there is an extensive list included at **www.neh.gov/grants/ listing?keywords=education.**
	Each entry has a due date and a project implementation date. The latter gives proposers the date by which they will be notified about funding.
Who is eligible	NEH grants typically go to cultural institutions, such as museums, archives, libraries, colleges, universities, public television, and radio stations, and to individual scholars.
Types of funding	According to the **1965 National Foundation on the Arts and the Humanities Act,** "The term 'humanities' includes, but is not limited to, the study of the following: language, both modern and classical; linguistics; literature; history; jurisprudence; philosophy; archaeology; comparative religion; ethics; the history, criticism and theory of the arts; those aspects of social sciences which have humanistic content and employ humanistic methods; and the study and application of the humanities to the human environment with particular attention to reflecting our diverse heritage, traditions, and history and to the relevance of the humanities to the current conditions of national life."
Process	Applicant for grants from the NEH must apply through **www.grants.gov** as is the case with many other government funding agencies. However, the NEH has its own grant funding management process with separate procedures for organizations and individuals. This can be found at **www.neh.gov/grants/ manage.**

TABLE 5.16. National Institutes of Health (NIH)

Website	www.nih.gov
Overview	The National Institutes of Health (NIH), a part of the U.S. Department of Health and Human Services, is the primary federal agency for conducting and supporting medical research to facilitate important medical discoveries that improve people's health and save lives. NIH scientists investigate ways to prevent disease as well as causes, treatments, and cures for both common and rare diseases. It is composed of 27 institutes and centers.
Finding funding	The NIH Guide for Grants and Contracts is the official publication for NIH medical and behavioral research grant policies, guidelines, and funding, at **http://grants. nih.gov/grants/guide/description.htm.** The NIH issues Funding Opportunity Announcements (FOAs) on a regular basis; these may be accessed at Grants.gov or through the link **http://grants.nih.gov.**
Who is eligible	Individuals—scientists at various stages in their careers, from predoctoral students on research training grants to investigators with extensive experience who run large research centers. However, there are special programs for new and early-stage investigators, who get special consideration and are eligible for programs targeting them. Institutions—in general, domestic or foreign, public or private, nonprofit or for-profit organizations are eligible to receive NIH grants.
Types of funding	The NIH is the largest source of funding for medical research in the world and funds thousands of scientists in universities and research institutions. Its institutes and centers each has a specific research agenda focused on particular diseases or body systems. These include cancer; eye; heart, lung, and blood; genome research; aging; alcohol abuse and alcoholism; allergies and infectious diseases; child health and human development; deafness and communication disorders; drug abuse; environmental health sciences; mental health; neurological disorders and stroke; and minority health and health disparities.
Process	Once you submit your proposal, it takes 1–3 months for the NIH to refer it for review. It then takes an estimated 4 months for peer review and 2 months for the pre-award process to be completed, with negotiations between NIH and the applicant followed by official notification of the applicant institution.

TABLE 5.17. National Science Foundation (NSF)

Website	www.nsf.gov
Overview	The NSF is the funding source for approximately 20% of all federally supported basic research conducted by America's colleges and universities. In many fields such as mathematics, computer science, and the social sciences, the NSF is the major source of federal backing. The NSF's goals—discovery, learning, research infrastructure, and stewardship—provide an integrated strategy to advance the frontiers of knowledge, cultivate a world-class, broadly inclusive science and engineering workforce, and expand the scientific literacy of all citizens.
Finding funding	The NSF site is very user friendly, and funding information can be found at **www.nsf.gov/funding.** The site offers the user the opportunity to search on special programs by type of student or by program areas.
Who is eligible	Each individual competition specifies eligibility. As a rule the following are eligible: college and university faculty and students, college–school partnerships, research laboratories, federally funded laboratories, unaffiliated and for-profit agencies and U.S. nonprofit research institutions. Each grant solicitation clearly states eligibility criteria, and the solicitations are organized so that this information is easy to find.
Types of funding	Student-related grants serve undergraduate, graduate, postdoctoral, and K–12 students or the following program areas: Crosscutting and NSF-wide, Biological Sciences, Computer and Information Science and Engineering, Education and Human Resources, Engineering, Environmental Research, and Education, Geosciences, International Science and Engineering, Mathematical and Physical Sciences, and the Social, Behavioral, and Economic Sciences.
Process	The NSF has its own process for grants submission, review, and notification called Fastlane. To have access to Fastlane, your organization must register with NSF as a Fastlane organization, and individuals must register as part of the organization. Proposals may also be submitted through Grants.gov.
Other information	The Proposal and Award Policies and Procedures Guide (PAPP) is a must-read document, as it provides guidance on proposal preparation and submission and award management.

TABLE 5.18. Annie E. Casey Foundation

Website	www.aecf.org
Overview	The Annie E. Casey Foundation is a private charitable organization dedicated to helping build better futures for disadvantaged children in the United States. It was established in 1948 by Jim Casey, one of the founders of UPS, and his siblings, who named the foundation in honor of their mother. The primary mission of the foundation is to foster public policies, human-service reforms, and community supports that more effectively meet the needs of today's vulnerable children and families. In pursuit of this goal, the foundation makes grants that help states, cities, and neighborhoods fashion more innovative, cost-effective responses to these needs. A fact sheet is accessible from the website.
Finding funding	In order to determine if your project meets the mission of the foundation you should review prior grants that the foundation has made. However, grant making of the Annie E. Casey Foundation is limited to grantees who have been invited by the foundation to participate in these projects. The foundation does not seek or often fund unsolicited grant applications, and in any given year, they have limited resources to fund additional, unsolicited proposals.
Who is eligible	If you are an educational or other institution, agency, or community organization you should determine, by reviewing the grants the foundation has awarded and the projects it conducts, if your mission is compatible. A sampling can be seen under the tabs Major Initiatives and Making Connections. If it is, let the foundation know about how your work might contribute to the success of its efforts.
Areas funded	The AECF uses its resources to partner with and forge collaborations among institutions, agencies, decision makers, and community leaders so they can work together to transform tough places to raise families by providing direct services, reforming public systems, providing strategic consulting, transforming neighborhoods, strengthening families, building economic success, using data and evaluation, and ensuring racial and ethnic equity.
Process	Write a letter to the foundation showing links between your work and the work they are doing, and where they are doing it.
Other information	The AECF publishes a variety of web-based reports available in the Kids Count area of their website. These include: *Early Warning! Why Reading by the End of Third Grade Matters,* and *2010 Kids Count State Education Indicator.*

TABLE 5.19. Carnegie Corporation of New York

Website	http://carnegie.org
Overview	Andrew Carnegie envisioned Carnegie Corporation as a foundation that would "promote the advancement and diffusion of knowledge and understanding." In keeping with this mandate, its work incorporates an affirmation of its historic role as an education foundation but also honors Andrew Carnegie's passion for international peace and the health of our democracy.
Finding funding	The Carnegie Corporation publishes abstracts of all its funded projects back to 1982 on its website, which contains a grant search tool. You can search for grants by program area, year, grantee, or amount. Each grant will return a record, which includes an abstract describing the purpose of the grant.
Who is eligible	Eligible entities include public agencies, universities, and public charities with a 501(c)(3).
Areas funded	The Carnegie Corporation provides grants for projects that fit within its funding priorities. It recommends that potential grant seekers study the programs section to familiarize themselves with program priorities. Under Urban and Higher Education for example, program areas include innovation: new designs for schools, colleges, and education systems; strengthening human capital; building knowledge and affecting policy; and opportunity equation.
Process	The Carnegie Corporation accepts letters of inquiry on a rolling basis and urges that representatives of organizations considering sending such a letter read the program description relevant to their project and review grants made in the area of interest before using the online submission form. Following a staff review, programs that meet the foundation's priorities may be contacted to submit a formal proposal.
Other information	Several initiatives of the Carnegie Corporation are of interest to seekers of education grants, as they provide an excellent resource for establishing need and for reviewing the literature in some areas of education. For example, "The Opportunity Equation: Transforming Mathematics and Science Education for Citizenship and the Global Economy," found at **www.carnegie.org/publications** (seach for Opportunity Education), is a good resource.

TABLE 5.20. Charles Stewart Mott Foundation

Website	www.mott.org/about.aspx
Overview	Through our programming, the foundation endeavors to enhance the capacity of individuals, families, or institutions at the local level and beyond in hopes that its collective work in any program area can lead to systemic change. The mission of the Charles Stewart Mott Foundation is to support efforts that promote a just, equitable, and sustainable society.
Finding funding	Once at the website, go to "seeking a grant." This will take you to an overview that will link you to information on what the foundation funds, what it does not fund, and limitations. This page also enables you to search by issue and region. It is suggested that you look at all the funding information and then determine if your program area is within its purview. For each area they show the last 10 grants issued.
Who is eligible	As is the case with other foundations, eligibility includes: 501(c)(3) organizations and units of government (schools and colleges). Other organizations are asked to submit an inquiry to the foundation.
Areas funded	The areas of funding are civil society, the environment, the foundation's Flint, Michigan, program, and pathways out of poverty. Each of the four programs has clearly stated guidelines, which you are encouraged to review before submitting a request for funding.
Process	Review the relevant issues and regions for funding. If you determine that your proposal meets their criteria based on program guidelines, geographic limitations, and funding limitations, complete an online letter of inquiry. They promise a reply within a few weeks.
Other information	The viewer is asked to provide feedback by rating each area of the website.

TABLE 5.21. ExxonMobil Foundation

Website	https://corporate.exxonmobil.com
Overview	The purpose of ExxonMobil's contributions program is to meet important community needs in ways that are compatible with its business interests. The foundation works with community agencies with which it has established relationships or with whom it proactively develops relationships.
Finding funding	The website details programs within each area of interest. You should review the areas in detail and determine which areas are most pertinent to your work. Some funding goes through professional organizations for training programs that may be of interest to the students you serve.
	Math/science outreach programs that encourage and motivate students and support the professional development of math and science teachers include the National Math and Science Initiative (NMSI); Mickelson ExxonMobil Teachers Academy; Bernard Harris Summer Science Camp; the Dream Tour; and the Sally Ride Science Academy. ExxonMobil works with many organizations to further their math/science priorities including the American Society for Engineering Education (ASEE); Junior Achievement; National Action Council for Minorities in Engineering (NACME); National Science Teachers Association (NSTA); Project NexT; Reasoning Mind; and the Science Ambassador Program.
Who is eligible	Eligible applicants include registered charities, nongovernmental organizations, and nonprofit educational, health-related, and cultural organizations and also educational institutions, professional organizations, school districts, strategic alliances (e.g., SECME), and minority scholarship organizations.
Areas funded	Community investment areas include education, with a particular focus on science and math and the education of women and girls; health, with a focus on improving public health and reducing health-related barriers to development in communities; and environment, focused on conserving biodiversity—the variety of life on earth.
Process	The website does not provide for an electronic letter of inquiry directly to the foundation. Since so much of its support for math and science is channeled through organizations listed in its program materials, networking with some of these programs might be a good way to begin to explore options.

TABLE 5.22. Ford Foundation

Website	**www.fordfoundation.org/Grants**
Overview	The foundation's grant making focuses on reducing poverty and injustice; promoting democratic values; and advancing human knowledge, creativity, and achievement.
Finding funding	It is critical to consult the funding database provided by the foundation to determine if your project fits its funding profile. It is searchable by regions, issues and initiatives, approaches, year, and amount of funding. It is a comprehensive resource that enables the viewer to roll the cursor over each grantee and see a brief description of the project. Clicking on the project provides information on how the project was categorized.
Who is eligible	Community organizations, institutions of higher education, charitable organizations, local educational agencies, school districts, professional associations, global development organizations, and almost any organization that is focused on the initiatives supported by the foundation.
Areas funded	The types of grants the foundation makes include project support, planning funding, competitive grants, matching funds, individual awards, endowment contributions, foundation-administered projects, and program-related investment.
Process	The Ford Foundation asks that applicants review areas of funding as well as previously funded project abstracts using the funding database before submitting grant inquiries using the online form found at **www.fordfoundation.org/work/our-grants/how-we-make-grants.**
Other information	The foundation provides a glossary of its grant-making approaches that is a must-read. It can be found at **www.fordfoundation.org/campaigns/grantmaking-glossary.** A good summary of the types of grant areas considered can be found at **www.fordfoundation.org/work/our-grants.**

TABLE 5.23. Gates Foundation

Website	**www.gatesfoundation.org**
Overview	The Gates Foundation lists 15 guiding principles in the opening section of the website, which, they indicate, "reflect the Gates family's beliefs about the role of philanthropy and the impact they want this foundation to have. The principles guide what we do, why we do it, and how we do it." They also describe their grant-making process as having four key steps: develop strategy, make grants, measure progress, and adjust strategy. Each of these steps is part of an overall continuing assessment process to assure that the foundation meets its goals and that the foundation learns from outcomes.
Finding funding	The website differentiates among three teams who oversee initiatives in the Global Development Program, the Global Health Program, and the United States Program. The U.S. program topics include Early Learning; Emergency Relief; High Schools; Libraries; Postsecondary Education; and Scholarships.
Who is eligible	Schools, school districts, educational associations, global development organizations, higher education institutions, professional associations, educational councils, and educational partnerships.
Areas funded	Common Core State Standards, college readiness for high school students, postsecondary success strategy, early learning, developmental education, effective teaching, and reducing inequity. Detailed information on these areas is at **www.gatesfoundation.org/How-we-work.**
Process	Sign on to **www.gatesfoundation.org** and review funding areas to apply for grants in global health and global development. Letters of inquiry are invited for some health-related areas. For U.S. education areas letters of inquiry are by invitation only.
Other information	The Gates Foundation Educational Strategy is detailed at **www.gatesfoundation. org/How-we-work** and is a "must read" before even thinking about contacting the foundation.

TABLE 5.24. IBM Community Foundation

Website	www.ibm.com/ibm/ibmgives
Overview	The primary focus of the foundation's corporate citizenship activities is on developing initiatives to address specific societal issues, such as the environment, community economic development, education, health, literacy, language, and culture. It employs IBM's most valuable resources, technology, and talent to create innovative programs in these areas to assist communities around the world.
Finding funding	In order to find specific areas for funding go to **www.ibm.com/ibm/ibmgives** and click on areas of interest to find additional information in each area. In education, for example, the areas include IBM KidSmart Early Learning Program; IBM MentorPlace; Reading Companion; Transition to Teaching; TryScience; Reinventing Education; and TryEngineering.
Who is eligible	Organizations that have a tax-exempt classification under Sections 170(c) or 501(c)(3) of the U.S. Internal Revenue Code.
Areas funded	The areas of interest for funding include education; adult training and workforce development; arts and culture; helping communities in need; and the environment.
Process	Grants are allocated to specific projects and programs that fit within IBM's targeted areas of interest. The overwhelming majority of funding activities are proactively initiated by IBM, and not a result of unsolicited proposals. The foundation does not encourage unsolicited proposals.
Other information	The IBM website has a library of reports related to its funding areas at **www.ibm.com/ibm/ibmgives.** These will be useful for individuals seeking grants from any funders.

TABLE 5.25. J. P. Morgan Chase

Website	www.jpmorgan.com/pages/jpmc/community/grants
Overview	J. P. Morgan Chase grants are focused in three areas: *Community development*— to address issues related to poverty and social exclusion by building economic infrastructure, promoting self-sufficiency, and supporting efforts to narrow social inequities; *Education*—to ensure that all children, particularly those from disadvantaged backgrounds, have access to high-quality educational opportunities with a particular focus on K–12 public schools that help them acquire the knowledge and skills needed to be productive, engaged citizens; and *Arts and culture*—to increase community access to rich cultural resources that foster creativity, promote self-expression, celebrate diversity, and strengthen our environment.
Finding funding	J. P. Morgan Chase is listed at the Foundation Center in a searchable database although there is a fee for use. For information on what types of organizations have been funded by Chase under various categories search on the website for funding. Also, Chase publishes an occasional community development newsletter that may be helpful in identifying the types of programs that are supported.
Who is eligible	This funder only funds 501(c)(3) charitable organizations. The specific limitations in its funding by type of organization, purpose, and location are provided on their web pages under "grant limitations."
Areas funded	Within each of the areas funded, there are specific areas of interest. In community development, funding is focused on workforce development, asset building, and financial literacy. For education funding Chase focuses on development of instruction leaders, implementation of innovative curricula, college access initiatives, deepening teacher content knowledge, and extending learning opportunities. In arts and culture Chase seeks to support arts programs in schools and after school, and build the capacity of community-based arts groups.
Process	The J. P. Morgan Chase grant application process begins with the submission of a letter of inquiry on the Grant Contacts page. Grant applications may be submitted throughout the year, but applicants are urged to contact the appropriate community representative (found listed by state at the website) before submitting a letter of inquiry. Applicants will be asked to provide information on the organization's mission, program/project description, program/project budget, and geography to be served, and your contact information. Once the letter of inquiry has been reviewed, you will be notified whether or not a full application is requested. If so, additional guidelines will be provided.

TABLE 5.26. Metropolitan Life Foundation

Website	www.metlife.com/corporate-responsibility/metlife-foundation
Overview	The MetLife Foundation was created in 1976 by MetLife to continue its long-standing tradition of contributions and community involvement. The goal is to empower people to lead healthy, productive lives and strengthen communities. Underlying the Foundation's programs is a focus on education at all ages and a commitment to increasing access and opportunity.
Finding funding	Finding funding at MetLife necessitates reviewing the areas and subareas in which the foundation gives the bulk of its funding and then determining which area includes your specific project idea. Look at past funding history to determine if MetLife has funded similar projects in past years. If so, continue to follow the process to determine if your organization is eligible.
Who is eligible	Uniquely, the MetLife Foundation offers an eligibility survey on its website to determine if the applicant is eligible to receive funding. The survey asks a series of questions to determine if the applicant is a 501(c)(3); U.S. based; and if you are a type of organization they do not fund. If you answer the all questions to their satisfaction, you are taken to the online application.
Areas funded	Areas and some of the subareas considered for funding by the MetLife Foundation include the following: health, including healthy aging and healthy habits; civic affairs, including urban neighborhood revitalization, after-school and mentoring programs and civic involvement; culture and public broadcasting, including access and inclusion in the arts, arts education, and public broadcasting; and education, an area that includes teaching and learning, and college access and success. The website provides detailed information on each area. Review of this is critical to determine if your project falls within the foundation's interests. MetLife also announces grants it has awarded.
Process	Requests are accepted and reviewed throughout the year. Requests and supporting materials are carefully evaluated by the MetLife Foundation. When an organization submits a request for either general or project support, both the organization and the proposal are evaluated.

TABLE 5.27. Pew Charitable Trust

Website	www.pewtrusts.org
Overview	The Pew Charitable Trust is driven by the power of knowledge to solve today's most challenging problems. Pew applies a rigorous, analytical approach to improve public policy, inform the public, and stimulate civic life. It partners with a diverse range of donors, public and private organizations and concerned citizens who share their commitment to fact-based solutions and goal-driven investments to improve society. Pew has three overarching areas of interest: *Improving public policy*—they study and promote nonpartisan policy solutions for pressing and emerging problems affecting the American public and the global community; *Informing the public*—the Pew Research Center, a Washington-based subsidiary, is home to most of the foundation's information initiatives. It uses impartial, fact-based public-opinion polling and other research tools to track important issues and trends; *Stimulating civic life*—Pew supports national initiatives that encourage civic participation. In its hometown of Philadelphia, it supports organizations that create a thriving arts and culture community and institutions that enhance the well-being of the region's neediest citizens.
Finding funding	The website has a database that enables a search of grants awarded by date, keyword or organization, or purpose.
Who is eligible	The majority of grants awarded by Pew are to public charities classified as tax exempt under section 501(c)(3) of the Internal Revenue Code.
Areas funded	The areas of funding are economic policy, the environment, health, and state policy and performance. Subareas include the following: *Health*: Public Health and Human Policy; Family Financial Security; and Science and Technology; *Environment*: Global Warming and Climate Change; Conservation of Living Marine Resources; and Old-Growth Forests and Wilderness Protection. The Pew Center on the States initiatives include Early Education, Partnership for America's Economic Success, Public Safety Performance Project, and Make Voting Work.
Process	The first step is to review the guidelines on the website; explore grants that have been awarded; review the descriptions of program areas; and submit a letter of inquiry that includes who, what, how and why, when, how much, and where. Your letter of inquiry will be reviewed by the appropriate staff. You will be notified in 4 to 6 weeks whether or not your request meets the funding criteria of the program.

TABLE 5.28. Robert Wood Johnson Foundation

Website	www.rwjf.org/grants
Overview	The Robert Wood Johnson Foundation provides grants for projects in the United States and U.S. territories that advance its mission to improve the health and health care of all Americans. For projects to be eligible for funding, they must address one of seven program areas. Visit each program area for more information on its strategic objectives and funding guidelines.
Finding funding	The foundation has useful detailed information about each of its funding areas (see below *), outlining its strategies and approaches. This information serves to define its goals and objectives in each area and gives information on what it has funded and what areas it plans to fund in the future. RWJ also posts information about previous funding—a good way to further determine if your project may be of interest.
Who is eligible	RWJ supports public agencies, universities, and public charities that are tax exempt under section 501(c)(3) of the Internal Revenue Code.
* Areas funded	The areas funded by the Robert Wood Johnson Foundation are Healthy Communities (Built Environment and Health, Disease Prevention and Health Promotion, Health Disparities and Social Determinants of Health); Healthy Children–Healthy Weight (Child and Family Well-Being, Childhood Obesity and Early Childhood); Health Systems (Health Care Coverage and Access, Health Care Quality and Value and Public and Community Health); and Leadership for Better Health (Health Leadership Development and Nurses and Nursing). The types of projects funded include service demonstrations; gathering and monitoring of health-related statistics; public education; training and fellowship programs; policy analysis; health services research and technical assistance; communications activities; and evaluations.
Process	The website has calls for proposals within each area with links to the process and specific information required.
Other information	The foundation shows overview of its strategies in each area. These overviews specifically indicate what it does and does not fund within each area. RWJ also enables interested researchers to sign up for e-mail alerts about new initiatives and new calls for proposals. **www.rwjf.org/en/how-we-work/grants-and-grant-programs.html.**

TABLE 5.29. Alfred P. Sloan Foundation

Website	www.sloan.org
Overview	The Sloan Foundation is unique in its focus on science, technology, and economic institutions. It believes the scholars and practitioners who work in these fields are chief drivers of the nation's health and prosperity. In each grant program, the foundation seeks proposals for original projects led by outstanding individuals or teams. The Alfred P. Sloan Foundation is interested in projects that will result in a strong benefit to society, and for which funding from the private sector, the government, or other foundations is not widely available.
Finding funding	The Sloan Foundation site lists six broad areas of interest. Under each broad area are subareas hot-linked to a description. By clicking on the Apply button in any of the sections you can determine whether funding is available, who to contact, and how to contact them.
Who is eligible	While the Sloan Foundation has no clear statement about eligibility, it can be inferred that individuals, institutions, community organizations, and businesses are eligible.
Areas funded	Among the projects funded by the Sloan Foundation are its research fellowships and the following: Digital Sky Survey; Encyclopedia of Life; Public Understanding of Science and Technology; Education and Careers in Science and Technology; Workplace, Work Force and Working Families; Awards for Excellence in Teaching Science and Mathematics; Information Technology and Dissemination of Knowledge; and Economic Institutions, Behavior and Performance.
Process	First visit the Sloan website to determine whether your project is in an area that the foundation supports. Each program description has an Apply button that will explain the availability of grants and whether unsolicited letters of inquiry are accepted. If you determine that letters of inquiry are accepted, submit a letter of inquiry (information is provided on the website regarding how to compose and submit an LOI). Those whose ideas are promising and fit into the scope of the foundation's work will be contacted and asked to submit a formal proposal. The grants page has guidelines on composing and submitting a formal grant proposal.
Other information	The Sloan Foundation offers a comprehensive overview at **https://sloan.org/grants/apply#tab-grant-proposal-guidelines** with links to funding resources including: grant making strategy, what we do not fund, the grant application process, letters of inquiry, grant proposal guidelines, grant forms and tips for writing a successful grant proposal.

TABLE 5.30. Rockefeller Foundation

Website	**www.rockefellerfoundation.org**
Overview	The Rockefeller Foundation concentrates on results and impact—the difference we make in lives, communities, and the world. The foundation fosters innovation in markets, organizations, products, and processes. It influences and informs public policy with cutting-edge ideas and research. It connects partnerships and networks, bringing people and institutions with diverse perspectives together across disciplines and sectors—and facilitating their learning from and with one another. It supports work that enables individuals, communities, and institutions to access new tools, practices, resources, services, and products. And it supports work that enhances their resilience in the face of acute crises and chronic stresses, whether manmade, ecological, or both.
Finding funding	Examples of the types of projects that the foundation funds are on its website in a searchable database. It encourages grant seekers to review previously funded projects and only if they believe the project to be submitted is within the foundation's purview, submit an online funding inquiry form.
Who is eligible	Individuals, communities, and institutions whose work builds on the areas of funding supported by the foundation.
Areas funded	The Rockefeller Foundation focuses its resources and energies on five interconnected issue areas that represent critical global challenges that the foundation is distinctively positioned to address: secure food, water, housing and infrastructure; accessible, affordable, and equitable health services and systems; sustainable growth and resilience in the face of climate change; solutions for fast-growing cities; and stronger safety nets, reinvigorated citizenship, and reimagined policy frameworks.
Process	The Rockefeller Foundation requests that you review descriptions of its work and funding initiatives, and if you have a project that fits within one or more of its funding areas you can submit an inquiry via its website. Proposals should not be sent unless invited by a member of the foundation staff in response to the funding inquiry form.
Other information	The Rockefeller Foundation offers links to other funders on its website as an additional resource for grant seekers at **www.rockefellerfoundation.org/grants/resources-grantseekers.**

TABLE 5.31. Spencer Foundation

Website	**www.spencer.org**
Overview	The Spencer Foundation funds research grants and fellowships in its mission to strengthen the connections among education research, policy, and practice and ultimately to improve students' lives and enrich society.
Finding funding	The Spencer Foundation website explicitly reviews the major areas of inquiry it aims to promote through its funding initiatives. By reading through the general information on the site, a potential applicant can quickly determine whether his or her research will fit into the precise areas of interest.
Who is eligible	Educational researchers at different stages of their professional careers and institutional initiatives aimed at improving the work and performance of agencies and institutions, primarily universities and graduate schools of education at universities.
Areas funded	The Spencer Foundation supports five areas of inquiry: education and social opportunity; organizational learning; teaching, learning, and instructional resources; purposes and values of education; and field-initiated proposals. Within each area the site provides detailed information in an overview containing a rationale for the area, relevant definitions, and questions of interest. A complete list can be found at **www.spencer.org/what-we-fund.** They also provide searchable summaries of the more than 5400 grants they have awarded at **www. spencer.org/grants.**
Process	The process of applying depends upon the type of funding being sought. The applicant should explore specific areas before beginning their proposal. In all cases all of the elements needed are outlined in detail on the website.
Other information	The Spencer Foundation has embarked on a grant effectiveness project to look at what types of research (Spencer and non-Spencer research) have influenced educational policy and practice, directly and indirectly, the type and level of the impact, and how the influence or impact evolved. The foundation issued a call for individuals to respond and has published the responses of 15 respected individuals on its website. It also publishes a bibliography of books and publications that have been funded wholly or partially by the Spencer Foundation. Information can be found at **www.spencer.org/archive/past-programs-projects/ mission-areas-of-inquiry.**

TABLE 5.32. Verizon Foundation

Website	www.verizon.com/about/responsibility/grant-requirements
Overview	The Verizon Foundation focuses its efforts on education and literacy and safety and health through innovative programs to improve literacy and strengthen education achievement for children and adults and by supporting initiatives to help prevent domestic violence and improve access to health care information and services.
Finding funding	Carefully read the information provided in each area the foundation supports and determine if your project meets their criteria by reviewing the funding goals and partnership guidelines. Also review the foundation's online sample grants. The foundation also suggests that you search for your community relations manager by entering your organization's zip code in the finder and that you contact him or her before applying or with any questions about the process. They may also be able to help you shape your idea so that it dovetails with foundation priorities.
Who is eligible	All qualified U.S.-based nonprofit organizations with a valid tax-exempt ID or 501(c)3 as well as public schools with a goal of assisting communities in the United States. In addition, the organization must be seeking funding in the areas of concern to the foundation.
Areas funded	The Verizon Foundation supports projects in the areas of: education and literacy (to improve literacy and strengthen educational achievement for children and adults by preparing them for success in the 21st century); domestic violence prevention (stop the violence before it begins with educational programs); health care and accessibility (invest in projects that provide technology to help underserved populations and people with disabilities access information on critical health issues as well as innovative technology that helps health care providers increase their efficiency, effectiveness, and reach); and Internet safety (proactively help people understand how to use the technology of the Internet safely).
Process	Once you determine that you are eligible (see quiz mentioned below), you must apply online as the foundation only accepts electronic proposals. It promises to acknowledge or respond to your application within 72 hours.
Other information	The Verizon Foundation has an eligibility quiz on its website that can be used to determine if a potential applicant is eligible. The site also provides access to guidance and examples for applicants so they understand what is required in their application. Under the tab Core Initiatives the foundation offers information on the areas it supports. This is critical reading to determine if your idea dovetails with theirs. Information can be found at **www.verizon.com/about/responsibility/grant-requirements**.

TABLE 5.33. W. K. Kellogg Foundation

Website	www.wkkf.org/grants
Overview	Our children are the world's future, and they depend on families, communities, and society at large to nurture and protect them, and to give them a platform for independence and success. But today, too many children grow up in a cycle of poverty that limits their access to adequate education, nutritious food, economic security, and quality health care. It's essential that we stand up for these children and change the social dynamics that hold some of them back. Kellogg is helping communities marshal their resources to assure that all children have an equitable and promising future.
Finding funding	As is the case with other foundations, WKKF has detailed information about each of its funding areas (see below), which is useful for applicants as they outline their strategies and approaches. It serves to define Kellogg's goals and objectives in each area and gives information on what it has funded and what areas it plans to fund in future. The foundation also posts information about previous funding, a good way to further determine if your project may be of interest.
Who is eligible	To be eligible for support, your organization or institution, as well as the purpose of the proposed project, must qualify under regulations of the United States Internal Revenue Service. As a result, WKKF is not able to provide funding directly to individuals.
Areas funded	The areas of interest are educated kids, healthy kids, secure families, racial equality, and civic engagement. As with some other foundations, Kellogg provides access to publications detailing strategies and goals within each of its areas of interest. Also provided are summaries of previously and currently funded projects, important information for a first time applicant to this or any foundation.
Process	If you believe your idea fits within the WKKF framework, please use the online application, which is how all requests for funding must be submitted. There are no submission deadlines. Grant applications are accepted throughout the year and are reviewed at corporate headquarters in Battle Creek, Michigan, or in Kellogg's regional office in Mexico (for submissions focused within their region).
Other information	WKKF publishes well-regarded information on project evaluation and on development of logic models for projects. A potential applicant would do well to review these documents before submitting even a preliminary proposal. In addition, the site provides compendiums of recent grants monthly.

PART II

Elements of the Proposal

CHAPTER 6

The Master Table and Creating Subtables

LEARNING OBJECTIVES

- What is a Master Table?
- Why create one?
- What elements should it contain?
- How do I create subtables?
- How do I estimate the cost of each program component?
- What is a fringe rate?
- What is an indirect cost?

I strongly recommend creating a Master Table for the proposal as you begin to write. The Master Table contains all information needed for all parts of the proposal and is used to create all other tables for the various sections of the proposal. The Master Table solves the all-too-frequent problem of having slightly different information in each of the proposal tables that has similar headings. This is off-putting to readers and can result in loss of score points critical to your placing in the funding band.

The column headings for the Master Table are Need, Objective, Activity, Description (of activity), Output, Outcome, Evaluative Measures, Responsible Personnel, Ambitious, and Attainable. If possible I would recommend that the table include project goals and budget information. Since the Master Table here contains budget numbers, some information on budget is presented in this chapter. However, Chapter 14 focuses on budget more comprehensively.

Table 6.1 includes column entries for each element under Project Goals 1, 1b, and 1c.

Table 6.2 shows how the cost of each activity was calculated. Form 6 at the end of the book is also downloadable and provides a template that the reader

TABLE 6.1. Master Project Table

Project Goal 1a: Increase the number/percent of low-income first-generation students completing 9th grade and entering 10th grade

Need	Objective	Activity	Ambitious	Attainable	Description	Output	Outcome	Evaluation	Staff	Budget
Low academic readiness for high school	95% of 9th-grade program students will be promoted to 10th grade each year.	Summer Bridge to High School (SBHS)	Currently fewer than 50% 9th-grade students are promoted to 10th grade. Transition to HS is the most critical stage of students' educational careers.	SBHS prepares students to function at a high school level during their freshman year and enables students to earn high school credits.	SBHS meets for 6 weeks in the summer for 6 hours a day; provides breakfast/lunch; enables students to earn up to 3 high school credits; provides instruction-/project-based learning in ELA, Math, and Science.	Students enter high school prepared to do high school work and with 1–3 high school credits.	90% of students perform better in their courses and earn sufficient credits to be promoted to 10th grade.	School and program attendance, GPA, earned credits, individual course grades, credits earned in SBHS, SAPR, and B/AST, Regents scores	Project coordinator, instructors, program adviser, group leaders, tutors	$46,997
		Saturday Academy Program (SAPR)	75% of high school 9th graders experience "9th-grade shock" and do not earn the credits needed to continue into 10th grade. Over 50% of students fail at least one course in 9th grade.	The SAPR provides review of work related to courses students are taking as well as the opportunity to earn additional credits.	SAPR meets on 10 Saturdays in the Fall and 10 Saturdays in the Spring for 6 hours each day; has individualized review and coursework; incorporates elements of the SBHS; enables students to earn HS credits.	Students can catch up; review difficult concepts; earn additional high school credits.			Project coordinator, instructors, program advisor, group leaders, tutors	$29,368
		Before/After-School Tutoring (B/AST)	75% of high school freshmen experience "9th-grade shock" and do not earn the semester	B/AST provides timely review of concepts and processes in the academic	B/AST meets 4 days per week before and after school. Solicits information from classroom teachers	Academic issues of students are addressed immediately				$19,840

			hours needed to continue into 10th grade. Over 50% of students fail at least one course in 9th grade.	areas in which students are experiencing confusion.	of participating students and uses marking period data to tailor tutoring for each student on an individual basis.	keeping them on track in their classes.		School and program attendance, GPA, earned credits	Project coordinator, instructors, program advisor, group leaders, tutors	Same as for Goal 1-SBHS and SAPR

Project Goal 1b: Increase the number of credits earned by low-income first-generation students entering 10th grade

More than 50% of 9th-grade students are held over because they do not earn sufficient credits for advancement to 10th grade.	90% of program students will have 10 or more credits by the end of 9th grade.	Summer Bridge to HS program / Saturday Academy Program (SAPR)	Currently fewer than 50% 9th grade students are promoted to 10th grade due to course failures during the 9th grade which reduce the number of credits earned.	SBHS/SAPR enables students to earn high school units during the summer and academic year that count toward promotion to 10th grade.	SBHS enables students to earn up to 3 high school units. SAPR enables students to earn additional HS credits on Saturdays.	Students can earn up to 6 credits toward the 10 needed for promotion to 10th grade.	90% of students earn sufficient credits to be promoted to 10th grade.	School and program attendance, GPA, earned credits	Project coordinator, instructors, program advisor, group leaders, tutors	Same as for Goal 1-SBHS and SAPR

Project Goal 1c: Increase the grade point average earned by low-income first-generation 9th-grade students

50% of student grades in the 9th grade are 65% or lower revealing a lack of subject matter mastery needed for continued success.	85% of program students will show an increase in GPA by 5% points by upper freshman term.	Before/After-School Tutoring (B/AST)	75% of high school freshmen experience "9th-grade shock" and do not master content/concepts required for further study. Over 50% of students fail at least two courses during the 9th grade.	B/AST provides timely review of concepts and processes in the academic areas in which students are experiencing confusion.	B/AST meets 4 days per week before and after school. Uses teacher and marking period data to tailor tutoring for each student on an individual basis.	Academic issues of students are addressed immediately keeping them on track in their classes.	85% of students increase their command of content knowledge and earn grades of 75 or better.	Program attendance, course grades, marking period and semester GPA, teacher assessment of student learning	Project coordinator, instructors, program advisor, group leaders, tutors	Same as for B/AST

95

TABLE 6.2. Figuring Out the Cost of Activities to Insert in Table 6.1

	Summer Bridge to High School	Saturday Academy Program	Before/After-School Tutoring
Project coordinator ($60,000)	24 days/365 in a year	20 days/365 in a year	
Site coordinators			4 schools × 20 weeks × 4 days × 2 hours × $25
Instructors	4 instructors × 6 weeks × 4 days × 5 hours × $50	4 instructors × 20 days × 4 hours × $50	4 instructors × 30 days × 2 hours × $50
Program adviser ($50,000)	24 days/365 in a year		
Group leaders	6 group leaders × 6 weeks × 4 days × 5 hours × $14	4 group leaders × 20 days × 4 hours × $14	
Tutors	6 tutors × 4 hours × 20 days × $12	4 tutors × 4 hours × 20 days × $12	4 tutors × 30 days × 2 hours × $12
Other than personnel costs	100 participants × $50	140 participants × $50	200 participants × $20
Indirect costs @ 8%	Total cost + 8%	Total cost + 8%	Total cost + 8%

can use. The project coordinator, with a full-time/annual salary of $60,000, earns $164.38 per day. Therefore the total salary allocated to the summer program is 24 days × $164.38. or, as shown in Table 6.3, $3,945. Please note that in budget submissions all totals are rounded to the nearest dollar. The required fringe benefit percentage for this full-time employee at my college is 33%, so the total benefits are $1,302. The total salary plus fringe attributable to the summer bridge program is $5,247. In similar fashion, the totals for each of the other cells in Table 6.1 are presented in Table 6.2. All the salaries and fringes are added together to determine the personnel costs for each program component.

All project budgets must include *"other than personnel"* costs and also have *indirect costs*. Form 7, a template which can be copied or downloaded for your use, is included at the end of the book. The other than personnel costs are all of the books and materials to be used by the program teachers and participants in the activity and must be accounted for in order to determine the cost of each component. The indirect rate recognizes the administrative costs to the organization/college for hosting the program. For our purposes we can use the indirect rate of 8%, which is the rate legislated for TRIO grants by the federal legislation. I have added this cost to each program component.

Now that you have a Master Table, you need to use it to create other tables for your proposal. For example, in the Evaluation section you need to present the Goal, the Objective, and the Evaluative Measures for the project. So you copy the entire table and delete all elements that are not needed, and produce a table for the evaluation section that consistently matches the contents of all other tables. Table 6.4 presents the extracted table that would be included in the evaluation section of your proposal. In similar fashion the Master Table can

TABLE 6.3. Budget Numbers and Total for Program Personnel across Three Activities

	Summer Bridge to High School	Saturday Academy Program	Before/After-School Tutoring
Project coordinator ($60,000) [33%]	$3,945 + $1,302	$3,288 + $1,085	
Site coordinators [10%]			$4,000 + $400
Instructors [10%]	$36,000 + $3,600	$24,000 + $2,400	$12,000 + $1,200
Program adviser ($50,000) [33%]	$3,288 + $1,085		
Group leaders [10%]	$2,016 + $202	$1,120 + $112	
Tutors [10%]	$1,728 + $173	$960 + $96	$3,840 + $384
Other than personnel costs	$5,000	$7,000	$4,000
Total component cost	$58,339	$40,061	$25,824
Indirect costs @ 8%	$4,667	$3,205	$2,066
Program activity total	$63,006	$43,266	$27,890

be used to create a table to demonstrate objectives and activities (Table 6.5); activities and descriptions (Table 6.6); and objectives, ambitious, and attainable (Table 6.7). Form 8 at the end of the book includes templates that you can copy or download to create the tables shown.

The Master Table *never* appears in the proposal but instead serves as the most up-to-date, accurate, unified, and comprehensive overview of your project/proposal. Any changes that are made to the project/proposal should be reflected in the Master Table, and once these changes are made the subtables created from this table are re-created. Working in this way assures that all tables in the proposal that have common information, such as percentages, number of days, number of students served, dates of service, budget numbers, responsible personnel, and the like are consistent. This is critical since the ultimate reader you are targeting is the external reviewer and discrepancies between and among tables in the proposal will result in the reader(s) losing confidence in the proposal as a whole even if the premise is excellent.

TABLE 6.4. Project Goal, Objective, and Evaluative Measures

Goal	Objective	Evaluative measures
Increase the number/percent of underrepresented students completing 9th grade and entering 10th grade.	90% of 9th-grade program students will be promoted to 10th grade each year.	School and program attendance; GPA; earned credits; individual course grades; credits earned in Summer Bridge to High School, Saturday Academy Program, and Before/After-School Tutoring; and Regents scores.

TABLE 6.5. Project Goal, Objectives, and Activities

Goal	Objectives	Activities
Increase the number/percent of underrepresented students completing 9th grade and entering 10th grade.	90% of 9th-grade program students will be promoted to 10th grade each year.	SBHS SAPR B/AST

TABLE 6.6. Project Activities and Descriptions

Activities	Descriptions
Summer Bridge to High School	Summer Bridge to High School meets for 6 weeks in the summer for 6 hours a day; provides breakfast/lunch; enables students to earn up to 3 high school credits; provides instruction/project-based learning in ELA, math, and science.
Saturday Academy Program	Saturday Academy Program meets on 10 Saturdays in the Fall and 10 Saturdays in the Spring for 6 hours each day; has individualized review and coursework; incorporates elements of the SBHS; enables students to earn high school credits.
Before/After-School Tutoring	Before/After-School Tutoring meets 4 days per week before and after school. Solicits information from classroom teachers of participating students and uses marking period data to tailor tutoring for each student on an individual basis.

TABLE 6.7. Objectives, Ambitious, and Attainable

Objectives	Ambitious	Attainable
90% of 9th-grade program students will be promoted to 10th grade each year.	75% of high school freshmen experience "9th-grade shock" and do not earn the semester hours needed to continue into 10th grade. Over 50% of students fail at least one course in 9th grade.	SBHS, SAPR, and B/AST assure readiness, enable students to earn high school credit, and provide timely review of concepts and processes in the academic areas in which students are experiencing confusion.

CHAPTER SUMMARY

Creation of a Master Table that does not appear in the proposal is recommended to assure that all tables presented throughout the proposal are consistent. The elements of the Master Table are Need, Objective, Activity, Description of Activity, Output, Outcomes, Evaluative Measures, and Responsible Individual. A Master Table for each project goal would be helpful. Budget allocations are also recommended if easily allocated by objective or by activity. The Master Table would be parsed into the various tables needed for other sections of the proposal. If changes have to be made to any table in the proposal, for example, if the percent of success has to be changed in objective(s), then it should be changed in the Master Table and then all tables reparsed for the proposal. A reader who encounters different information in different tables for the same item will question the accuracy of the whole proposal.

CHAPTER 7

Narrative Summary of Proposal Elements

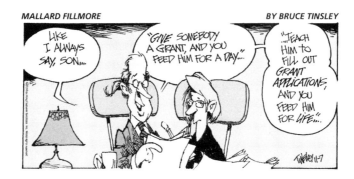

MALLARD FILLMORE   BY BRUCE TINSLEY

LEARNING OBJECTIVES

- How do I begin drafting my proposal?
- What sections should I include in my proposal and how should I format them?
- What points are awarded for each section of my proposal?
- What information should each section of my proposal contain?

The first materials I put on paper as I begin to think about and draft my proposal are the formatting guidelines, the due date, the submission website, and the selection criteria. These selection criteria with all subcriteria and the point values serve as my table of contents and an outline for the proposal I will write. I also do not write the proposal in selection criteria order. Rather, I jump around and fill in information I know and create the tables I know I will need in each section (at least in outline form). Also, since I have written so many proposals in my working life (over 500 and I have saved every one of them electronically), I have a lot of table templates to bring into the draft proposal.

The sections to be included in any proposal are specified in the RFP released by the agency. More important, however, is the fact that the RFP often indicates the points that are to be awarded for each section. This set of selection criteria is provided to the proposal readers, who use them to score

An example of a set of guidelines with point values is provided in Figure 17.1. It should be noted that the sequence presented here is generic. All RFPs that contain selection criteria have specific wording and subheadings and in all cases should be used as the outline for your proposal. In the chapters that follow, each selection criterion is addressed in detail with suggestions on how to approach the writing of the section.

You should view the proposal narrative as a series of events connected by a cause-and-effect system or sequential relationship. Each section is written to follow the sequence in the proposal guidelines and provide the requested information, and each section contains the information that supports the material or approach provided in the following section. Practice exercises for each proposal section are presented after Chapter 18.

You will see, for example, that the first narrative section, detailed below, introduces your project and provides an overview of your institution and why you are best qualified to serve your target population. The next section is need for the project, followed by goals and objectives. These goals and objectives lead to the activities that will address the needs you identified. The Plan of Operation is the *schedule of implementation* for the activities to assure that objectives are accomplished, including *procedures, management, key personnel,* and *timeline*. Finally, the evaluation section ties together the goals and objectives with the assessments and measurement that will reveal whether the project has achieved its purpose. The budget should reflect the scope of the proposal and should relate to the activities, personnel, number of participants, and timeline. A budget narrative briefly explains the elements and costs in the budget so that the reader understands how the budget is linked to the personnel and activities of the project.

You should:

- Make sure that your purpose and goals reflect those in the RFP.
- Complete only what the funding agency requires!
- Read the guidelines carefully and be concerned with every detail.
- Look for clues or keywords that will enhance the proposal.
- Provide documentation wherever necessary—this is essential.
- Support statements made in the narrative with background information, data, and other appropriate and reliable terminology.

The proposal narrative includes:

- Abstract or summary
- Introduction or background
  - Institutional expertise
- Statement of need or problem
- Objectives and/or goals of the project

- Plan of Operation
  - Activities to be conducted
  - Procedures for conducting the research/project
  - Management/organization of project
  - Key personnel and qualifications
  - Timeline or chart with the schedule for project implementation/ completion
- Evaluation procedures
- Dissemination strategy (if needed)
- Sustainability plan (if needed)
- Budget

Abstract or Summary

The abstract should be written first and reviewed and modified as needed. It presents the nature, scope, and outcomes for the project. Your relationship to the project is included as well as an indication of the overall cost of the project. Each agency will have specific guidelines for what needs to be included in the abstract. Often they want a one-page abstract that can be published on the website if you are funded.

Introduction or Background

The Introduction explains the subject being dealt with in the proposal. Background and support documentation must be included. At this point you establish credibility as an applicant for funding. You provide your background, training, related or previous research, accomplishments, and general goals. It is a good idea to begin the introduction by showing your proposal's relationship to the issues and concerns that are highlighted in the RFP.

Statement of the Need or Problem

The Statement of Need or Problem indicates why this project is being proposed. It may not be obvious to the reviewer that there is a need, and the applicant must establish it based on evidence and references that a need, in fact, exists.

Goals and Objectives of the Project

The specific and realistic goals of the project are presented. This section may include global goals with specific objectives. It is useful to organize the objectives according to the goal each set is designed to accomplish. If the needs/

problems are well defined, each goal/objective can be linked to the need it addresses. This makes it easier for the readers to see how your project relates to the need it is designed to address. Goals describe future expected outcomes and provide programmatic direction. They focus on ends rather than means. Objectives are clear, realistic, specific, measurable, and time-limited. There are two types of objectives: process objectives, which specify the means to achieve the outcomes, and outcome objectives, which address the results to be obtained.

Plan of Operation

The Plan of Operation contains several important subsections. This section allows the applicant to present how he or she will pursue the project. It includes the procedures and what is being utilized or applied in the project. An indication of what this methodology will accomplish that others haven't or won't is essential. How do you know that this activity or set of activities will lead to realization of the objectives? I generally use a table that links the goals, objectives, and activities to the individuals/staff with the responsibility for conducting/monitoring them.

• *Activities to be conducted.* Use tables that show the relationship between goals, objectives, activities, and evaluation measures.

• *Procedures for conducting the research/project.* Management/organization of project

• *Organizational chart.* Use an organizational chart for your institution and show how the project fits into the existing structure. (Some agencies indicate to whom the project director should report.)

• *Key personnel and qualifications.* Who are the key individuals in your organization that will oversee the project? What are their qualifications? What have they done previously? What will be their specific responsibilities with regard to the project? If they will still be in their current job, what percent of time will be allocated to the project? The résumés of all critical individuals should be included in an appendix. The use of a table here is also helpful.

• *Timeline for project completion.* Use of a timeline or chart to demonstrate how the activities and accomplishments of your project will be sequenced indicates that you have thought about and considered when events should occur and how long they will take. Also important to include is who will be responsible for completion of the activities and who will be responsible for seeing that the timelines are followed.

Evaluation Procedures

The Evaluation Procedures section provides an indication of how the project will be assessed to determine its success or achievement of the objectives. This section should be tied directly to the stated objectives and may include who will review the project, outside evaluation methods, data to be collected, research protocols, if any, to be used, and how the evaluation will be used to modify and improve the project. Both formative and also summative evaluation processes should be used for all funded projects.

Dissemination Strategy

Dissemination means informing others about the results of the project or research and most especially highlighting what has been learned from the project/research in the way of best practices. The degree of emphasis placed on dissemination in the proposal is dependent upon the guidelines of the funding agency and the type of project. A published report or article may be necessary. Perhaps regional or local workshops are to be given. A manual or guide for curriculum may be sent to teachers. The funders want to support change within communities and within institutions, and sharing the results of your project helps to broaden the impact of your work.

Dissemination may be accomplished in one or more of the following ways and should include plans to provide information through a project website:

Conferences	Presentations
Curriculum guides	Pamphlets
Seminars	Books or manuals
Newsletters	Audiovisual materials
On-site visits for professionals	Model courses or curricula
Media releases	Inservice training programs
Working papers	Self-instructional materials
Articles in journals	Demonstrations of techniques

Dissemination is an often overlooked or poorly developed section. Often it is treated as a throwaway section written last and without much thought. It adds value to the proposal and will show the readers/granting agency that thought has been given to how the grant findings will support change in the community and inform a broad constituency about the implications/best practices of the program. Dissemination helps broaden the impact of the funds that are being invested in your work.

A proactive dissemination strategy will assure outreach to multiple audiences in ways that will influence attitudes and behavior. This section might list relevant conferences and journals where this work will be presented and how materials developed by and for the project will be made available to others within the institution and to other institutions. For example, it might be stated that the curriculum and project-based learning modules will be available on the project website and through CDs that may be requested by others.

Sustainability Plan

Most funders want to know that the work they have supported will continue after funding ends. Sustainability might be considered to be synonymous with institutionalization. For grants such as the DHHS Strengthening Institutions (e.g., Title III, Title V), a request for new funding must focus on new needs, goals, and objectives and, if applicable, should show how previously funded efforts have been sustained/institutionalized.

In many cases sustainability means that an institution will maintain and continue aspects of the project using institutional funds. This might include continuing to employ project advisors, continuing to pay for software packages that provide early warning for student performance, continuing to fund tutoring and other student support services, and institutionalizing activities that increase student retention and graduation.

Budget

A typical budget will have three sections: personnel, "other than personnel" expenses, and indirect costs.

- Personnel related
  - Salaries
  - Fringe benefits
- Non-personnel related
  - Space (facilities)
  - Equipment
  - Materials and supplies
  - Travel
  - Telephone
  - Other (postage, printing, fees, etc.)
- Indirect costs

CHAPTER SUMMARY

The narrative summary of proposal elements is drawn from the selection criteria presented in the RFP. It is suggested that the full selection criteria be used as your table of contents and proposal outline. Information on the contents of each section is described as well as possible, using figures, tables, and charts needed to clarify the narrative.

CHAPTER 8

Preparing the Abstract and Introduction

LEARNING OBJECTIVES

- What should an abstract for a proposal contain?

- How can I find good examples of abstracts?

- When should I write the abstract?

- What is the purpose of the introduction?

- What information should an introduction contain?

- How important is the introduction?

Abstract

The abstract should be written first and should be carefully reviewed and edited after the proposal is complete. As the first element you write, it provides an overview of your early vision of the project and can guide your planning and thinking. An abstract presents the nature, scope, and outcomes for the project. Your relationship to the project is included as well as an indication of the overall cost of the project. Each agency will have specific guidelines for what needs to be included in the abstract. Often they want a one-page abstract that can be published on the website if you are funded.

Most funding agencies will publish abstracts of funded projects online. This is a good way for you to read abstracts of successful proposals and get a comprehensive overview of how successful proposals briefly present their projects.

In some cases the RFP will specify what should be included in the abstract. For example, the RFP for a recently submitted proposal suggested:

> The abstract is limited to one page, single spaced. The abstract should describe the target area to be served, the services that will be provided and the activities to be conducted during the 5-year performance period. It should also include the citations, if applying for competitive priority points.

For a recent Upward Bound competition, it was suggested:

> All applicants must provide a one-page abstract. Complete instructions for submitting the abstract are included in the Instructions for Completing the Application Package in this application. The abstract must be uploaded into the *ED Abstract Form* in Grants.gov.

In Grants.gov, the abstract has the following text:

> The abstract narrative must not exceed one page and should use language that will be understood by a range of audiences. For all projects, include the project title (if applicable), goals, expected outcomes and contributions for research, policy, practice, etc. Include population to be served, as appropriate. For research applications, also include the following:
>
> - Theoretical and conceptual background of the study (i.e., prior research that this investigation builds upon and that provides a compelling rationale for this study).
> - Research issues, hypotheses and questions being addressed.
> - Study design including a brief description of the sample including sample size, methods, principal dependent, independent, and control variables, and the approach to data analysis.

In the abstract you have to say a lot in a few words, so the editing process is most important here. As this is the reader's first introduction to your project, it should include elements of the need for the project, distinguishing features of your approach, outcomes you will achieve, how you will attain them, and the measures you will use to evaluate project accomplishments. Practice exercises are presented after Chapter 18.

Introduction

The introduction explains the issue dealt with in the proposal. The introduction has to convince the reader that your proposal addresses an important issue and that your institution or organization has the knowledge, resources, and skills to follow through with an action plan that leads to one or more sustainable solutions. The introduction sets the stage, so to speak, for the rest of the proposal. It seizes the reader's attention and draws him or her into the argument and solution you are offering.

The introduction enables the applicant to establish his or her credibility for funding. It is useful to view the introduction as a marketing proposal in which you are "selling" or "positioning" your institution as the best possible choice for successfully carrying out this project. In writing the introduction, you must incorporate the purpose as stated in the RFP as central to your institution by framing any information you include in the words of the RFP.

- What is the mission/vision of the institution?

- How does the RFP purpose enable the institution to meet specific needs of the institution, its students, and/or the community?

- What is the innovative idea that undergirds your request for funding?

- How do the characteristics of the institution match the qualifications stated in the RFP?

- What are the elements that uniquely prepare the applicant for achieving the goals and objectives of the RFP?

- What has the applicant achieved recently that shows the capability of guiding the project to successful outcomes?

- What is the literature/research you have consulted that supports your innovative idea, the goals and objectives you have set, and the outcomes you expect?

In your institution you should be able to find materials that have been prepared for accrediting agencies (Middle States, CAEP) in response to strategic planning for the future; for college mission and vision statements; for furthering community commitments and partnerships; and/or for presidential reports on the state of the college and its future.

Institutional background and support documentation must be included. The applicant should highlight background, training, related or previous research, accomplishments, and general goals. It is a good idea to begin the introduction by showing the relationship of the proposal to the issues and concerns highlighted in the RFP. Practice exercises are presented after Chapter 18.

CHAPTER SUMMARY

This chapter dealt with the abstract and the proposal introduction. These sections must be written in a way that grabs the reader's attention and piques his or her interest in your proposal. The abstract is often used when listings of funded proposals are posted on the funder's website. While the abstract is written first, frequent review and editing are recommended to assure that it provides an accurate summary of the project. Most funders specify what should be contained in the abstract, and although it is not scored, following the outline will help readers to easily compare the many proposals they read. The introduction provides the reader with the first view of the applicant and enables the applicant to establish institutional/organizational credibility in relation to the proposal to be presented. In the introduction you are, for the first time, selling or positioning your institution as the best possible choice for achieving the goals and objectives proposed.

CHAPTER 9

An In-Depth Look at Logic Models

LEARNING OBJECTIVES

- What is a logic model?

- What are the elements/headings that are addressed in a logic model?

- Where can I find resources on creating logic models?

- What does a logic model look like?

- How should I go about formulating a logic model?

When I began writing proposals I had a mentor who urged me to think about how to show the relationships among the parts of my proposal so that the readers could understand that the need was related to the goals and the objectives I set were integral to achieving those goals and the objectives led to the activities I chose to implement. Further, the activities were related to the outcomes that I measured and looped back to the achievement of the initial objectives I had proposed to address the needs I had identified at the outset.

My response to this was to create tables such as the Master Table presented in Chapter 6. In truth, this Master Table was a version of a logic model without the preferred headings that are now recommended to systematize its use.

Many funders are now asking proposers to use a logic model as a framework for presenting and describing the relationships between and among program resources, program design, individuals served, outcomes, and short-term and long-term results. It is a way to chart the course of your project and is closely tied to effective project evaluation. Frequently, a logic model is viewed as an approach to integrating planning, implementation, evaluation, and reporting. There are many links to logic model development websites provided in Appendix B but let's review the basics.

It should be noted that some people find logic models repetitive because the information there is often contained in other parts of the proposal and is simply a restatement of the obvious. This repetition is OK because you are writing the proposal for the reader who needs and wants an overall picture of your project for reference in reading your proposal. Presenting the same information in different ways can provide detail and clarity about your project. Practice exercises are included after Chapter 18.

What Is a Logic Model?

What Is a Logic Model?

It is a systematic, visual way to show the relationships among project resources, activities, and results you hope to achieve. Most simply, it is a project road map comprised of project resources, activities, outcomes, and short- and long-term impacts.

A logic model links outcomes and short-term and long-term impacts with program resources, activities/ processes, and the theoretical assumptions/principles of the program. It is a systematic, visual way to show the relationships among project resources, activities, and results you hope to achieve. Most simply, it is a project road map, detailing a sequential chain of if–then relationships among the steps of a project that illustrates the connections among its elements. A very basic logic model consists of assumptions based on theory, research, evaluation, and knowledge that support the premises of your project and external factors or variables that need to be taken into account in conducting the project.

Specific components include inputs (the resources to be used in the project and the activities to be implemented) and outputs (the project outcomes and the short- and long-term impacts that will result). We use implicit logic models every day in making and carrying out decisions.

One of the best guides to developing logic models is available from the W. K. Kellogg Foundation and is online at **www.wkkf.org/-/media/pdfs/log-icmodel.pdf.** This is the most often used and widely disseminated resource. There are several other resources that can assist in thinking about and developing logic models. The most useful interactive logic model resource is from the University of Wisconsin Extension, at **https://fyi.uwex.edu/program-development/logic-models,** and provides a link to an online course as well as a static printable version of the interactive online course. Those who have the time will greatly benefit from actually working through the course, which is very helpful and informative. Chapter 13, on evaluation, will refer back to logic models as a useful tool in designing your proposal evaluation.

Why Use a Logic Model?

Many funders now ask that the proposal explicitly contain a logic model to illustrate how the elements of the project lead to immediate, short-, and long-term outcomes. Creation of a logic model requires systematic, critical thinking about the components of your project and the relationships between and among them. It provides an opportunity to work with colleagues to create a step-by-step progression and sequence for the work and to see how well the components fit together. Review and modification of the logic model affords the project development team chance to think through the process. Use of a logic model helps to find inconsistencies in the sequence of a program, creates an understanding of the program and how the components work together, spotlights connections between action and results, and reveals how well the evaluation captures outcomes. The Master Table introduced in Chapter 6 that details the relationships among project objectives, activities, outcomes, evaluation measures, and responsibilities is similar to a logic model but does not include the necessary components of resources and short- and long-range impacts.

Logic Model Basics

A logic model is a visual representation of a series of if–then assumptions. If the program has the needed resources, then you can use them to implement the activities you have planned for the project. If you implement the activities as planned, then the project participant outcomes will be as you have predicted. If these outcomes are achieved, then certain measureable changes

> **Logic Model Basics**
>
> A logic model visually presents an if–then model for your project. It is a sequential and connected representation of how your project elements are connected and related.

will occur. If the outcomes are achieved, then short- and long-term impacts will result and your project will be successful. The program components of the logic model include resources/inputs, participants, activities, outcomes, and impacts.

The resources/inputs are elements that can facilitate or impede program effectiveness. Factors that can facilitate a program are funding, collaborators, existing relationships, equipment, space, and supplies. Factors that can impede a program can include lack of space, poor attitudes, organizational limitations, and regulations. The target population is part of the resources/input of the logic model and can be characterized by age, ethnicity, income, and other demographic factors.

The activities are the components of the program and can include course curricula, educational strategies, computer programs, training programs, counseling, and career and other workshops designed to bring about the desired effects.

The outputs are comprised of the services delivered or products produced. These may be most closely linked to formative assessment. Did the program serve the number of planned participants? Were the intended workshops offered? Was the demographic profile of the participants as intended? Was the time schedule as expected?

The short- and long-term impacts are specific results or measureable outcomes that can be linked to the program activities. They are comprised of organizational, community, and/or system-level changes that may result from the inputs and program activities.

Examples of logic models are presented in Table 9.1 and Figures 9.1 and 9.2. If you have access to a program like Smart Draw or to a graphics professional, you can create logic models that look like the example presented in Figure 9.2.

TABLE 9.1. Simple Logic Model for Increasing Academic Attainment in College

Inputs	Activities	Output	Short-term impact	Long-term outcomes
• Low-income first-generation students • Transition advisers • Academic advisers • Data analysts • Peer mentors/tutors • Career/academic advisers • Counselors • Faculty • Financial support • Library workshops	• Provide transition advising • Transfer events • Major events • Enhance course offerings • Professional development for faculty and staff • Develop articulation • Courses offered winter/summer	• No. of students using support services • No. of students participating in co-curricular activities • No. of students meeting with transition adviser and no. of meetings • No. of students completing degree profile • No. of students completing long-range academic plan • No. of community college transfer events & no. of students attending • No. of major events offered and no. of students attending • No. of courses offered winter/summer	• Increase no. of contacts students have with advisers (Obj. 2.5) • Increase student awareness of transfer, major, and career options, course offerings, and of their status • Increase student grades in first major course by 5%/year (Obj. 1.3) • Increase number of credits earned by participating students 3%/year (Obj. 1.2) • Increase credits earned each semester and year by 3% (Obj. 4.1) • Increase fall-to-spring persistence of students by 3% (Obj. 2.1) • Increase fall-to-fall persistence of students by 3% (2.2) • Increase no. of students who complete 24–30 credits each year by 1% (Obj. 1.4)	• Increase percentage of participating students who declare a major with 45–60 credits by 4% (Obj. 2.4) • Increase GPA of participating students by 3% each year (Obj. 1.1) • Increase overall second- to third-year persistence of students by 3% (Obj. 2.3) • Increase no. of students who earn AA-AAS degrees in 2 years by 2% (Obj. 4.2) • Increase no. of students who earn BA degrees in 4 years by 2% (Obj. 4.3) • Increase percentage of students who graduate within 6 years by 5% (Obj. 4.4)

Inputs	Activities	Outcomes	Short-Term Impact	Long-Term Impact
Community college partners (Bronx and Hostos)	**Social Capital Intervention:** • Combination of social belonging and difference education evaluation	No. who complete the social capital intervention	**PM1:** Significantly greater sense of belonging for treated versus control group students *immediately* following intervention	**PM2:** Significantly higher STEM retention/graduation rates for STEM treatment versus control group students by September 2021
Lehman faculty Lehman staff and programs	**Social Support Innovations:** • Intrusive advising • Academic support services (e.g., tutoring) • Guaranteed admission agreement	No. who complete (a) guaranteed admission agreement and (b) financial aid requirements; no. who attend (a) advising, (b) support services, and (c) workshops; no. of advisement sessions held, workshops developed	Increased (a) understanding of STEM academic and career choices, (b) self-efficacy, (c) identity as a scientist, (d) research skills, and (e) perceptions of support from STEM community	By September 2021, 10% increase in students: **PM3:** Seeking STEM degree **PM4:** Completing 2-year degree within 3 years **PM5:** Transferring to a 4-year from a 2-year college in STEM
Guest speakers Time and money	**Instructional Innovations:** • Academic strategies (e.g., summer classes) • Research experience • Faculty professional development (PD)	No. who participate in (a) faculty PD, (b) academic innovations/strategies, (c) research experiences, and (d) externships; creation of STEM resource center and webpage	Increased GPA and progress toward graduation Increased faculty collaboration and implementation of instructional innovations	**PM6:** Retained in STEM **PM7 and PM8:** Graduated in STEM within 3 years (transfer); 6 years (freshmen)
	Curriculum Innovations: • AS in Liberal Arts and Science • STEM articulation agreements with Bronx Community College	No. of STEM tracks, concentrations, and certificate programs developed; students who enroll in programs	Increased no. of students (a) pursuing STEM programs at Bronx Community College and Lehman and (b) maximizing credits accepted in transfer; increased student satisfaction with STEM programs and transfer process	

FIGURE 9.1. Logic Model for the Pathways to Student STEM Success (PTS³) program at Lehman College.

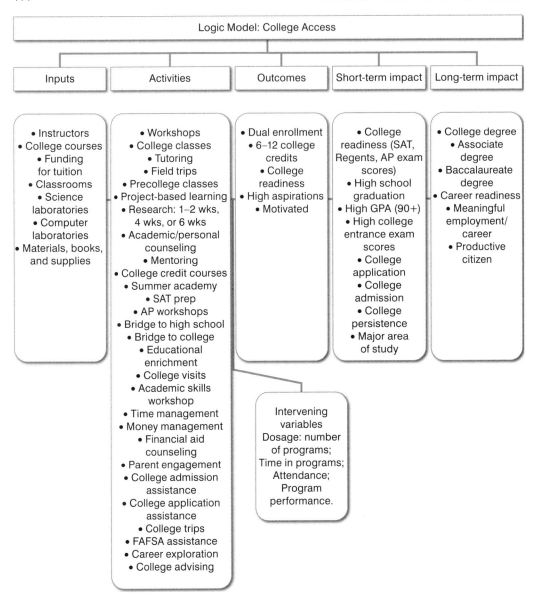

FIGURE 9.2. Logic model for college access/readiness proposal.

Logic Model Exercise

The logic model exercise takes advantage of the consensus project that was fully described in Chapter 2, so only highlights of the process are included here. Gather individuals with a vested interest in the project who understand the overall purpose of the RFP (based on a summary you have provided) and of what you are trying to accomplish for your likely participants (needs you are addressing).

1. Before starting your logic model, prepare several large sheets of paper with the following headings (each on an individual sheet):
   - Inputs/Resources
   - Activities
   - Outcomes
   - Short-Term Impact
   - Long-Term Impact

2. Bring:
   - 3″ × 5″ sticky notes
   - The RFP
   - Project goals statement
   - Project objectives

3. Provide the sticky notes to the group you have assembled and ask them to answer, in turn, the following questions:
   - What will the participants served by this project know and be able to do at the end of the project (outcome)?
   - What activities will enable participants to achieve these outcomes?
   - What resources will be needed to conduct these activities for these participants?
   - What are the short-term impacts we can expect?
   - What are the long-term impacts we can expect?
     - Each member of the group uses one sticky note for one item to answer the specific question.
     - Each member in turn posts his or her sticky notes in turn.
     - The first member posts each different item in a separate column.
     - The following members post their sticky note in the column it most aligns with.
     - If there is no alignment, the member starts a different column.
     - Once all sticky notes are posted, each set of unique outcome notes should be consolidated into one agreed-upon outcome and written on the outcome sheet.

4. Once you have completed your sticky note chart and transferred the agreed-upon items to the charts, you have an initial workable logic model.

Logic Model Uses

The logic model provides an overall picture of the phases of the project and can be used to produce a focused description of what you are trying to accomplish. It can help in preparing the abstract. The resources you identify can be used to create a section on what the organization will contribute to the project. The activities and outcomes will be used in the Plan of Operation where you will describe what you will do, how you will do it and when. The short- and long-term impacts that you pose will become the heart of your evaluation section and will help you to create meaningful project goals and objectives. Finally, the outcomes will enable you to create a picture of how participants in your project will change and grow as a result of your intervention.

The logic model also has the benefit of showing the scope of the project on one page in a sequential and meaningful way. This can be used by project staff at regular meetings to assure that the project is on track. It can be used to focus new hires on the elements and connectedness of the project elements. If you have an outside evaluator, it will be created with his or her help and assure that the evaluation measures are consistent with what you aim to accomplish. Finally, the logic model can be used to determine the level of agreement with project aims among colleagues and modified if needed.

The more detail included in the logic model the better it can be used to follow the progress of the project. A detailed model can be used to prepare project reports, drive discussions at project meetings, review the progress of the project, and determine if the outcomes you proposed were realized.

CHAPTER SUMMARY

Many RFPs require a logic model as part of your proposal narrative. The Master Table discussed in Chapter 6 is somewhat akin to a logic model, but the funders are looking for a specific structure in a logic model. While some think the logic model is redundant, it serves a specific purpose by requiring all applicants to use a similar format to provide an overview of the reasoning behind their proposal. Readers can see the thinking that is behind the organization of the proposal. Perhaps more important, the proposers can reflect on how the available resources contribute to the achievement of objectives through the specific activities and how the activities lead to the short-, mid-, and long-term outcomes. Links to web-based resources on Logic Models and Logic Model exercises are included to assist you with developing a useful model for your projects.

Establishing Need for the Project

To illustrate the process of establishing need for a project, I am using the selection criteria for the TRIO Regular Upward Bound project as published in *Electronic Code of Federal Regulations* (Title 34, Part 645, Subpart 31). Selection criteria for this and other funded programs are made available in the *Federal Register* when the RFP is published and proposals are solicited. They are also included in the application guidelines that can be downloaded from the USDE website for the specific program.

(a) Need for the project (24 points). In determining need for an Upward Bound project, the Secretary reviews each project using the need criteria specified in this section. The maximum score for the need section is 24 points and selection criteria are as follows:

(1) The Secretary evaluates the need for a Regular Upward Bound project in the proposed *target area* on the basis of information contained in the application which clearly demonstrates that—

(i) The income level of families in the *target area* is low;

(ii) The education attainment level of adults in the *target area* is low;

(iii) Target high school dropout rates are high;

(iv) College-going rates in target high schools are low;

(v) Student/counselor ratios in the target high schools are high; and

(vi) Unaddressed academic, social and economic conditions in the *target area* pose serious problems for low-income, potentially first-generation college students.

Any proposal you submit must address each of the selection criteria in detail; in this case, you must use the exact language of each item as the title of subsections i–vi. As the number of pages is limited, the title of the section can be abbreviated as "(a) Need for the project" and statement 1 need not be included. Use an *italic font* (as above) in order to set the exact criteria apart from your text. The subsections i–vi should be numbered exactly as in the criteria.

The first step is to determine what types of data you need to show that the statements are true for your target population. For criteria i and ii, the data can be found online through the United States Census Bureau's American FactFinder site (**https://factfinder.census.gov**). The RFP indicates that the TRIO programs define "low income" as 150% of the poverty level and include the current U.S.-defined poverty level in their application materials. Of course, American FactFinder does not provide exactly the number and percentage you need, so you have to do some interpolation of the data. Table 10.1 and the explanation below provide an example of how to determine the precise information.

The federal poverty level for 2016 is reported online at **https://familiesusa. org/product/federal-poverty-guidelines** as $24,300. We can also determine from this same chart that for a family of 4, 150% of poverty equals an income of $36,450. American Factfinder results for the Bronx indicate that 484,902 individuals have incomes at 150% of poverty. This is 34% of the population of the Bronx. However, the RFP asks for families. Unfortunately, the chart does not specifically indicate poverty levels for families but provides ranges. Thus, we have to interpolate to find the specific percentage of families

TABLE 10.1. Demographic Profile for Bronx County, New York, Showing Poverty Levels for Determining 150% of Poverty Level

	Individuals		Families	
Total number	484,902	± 1.71	319,265	± 2,640
Less than $10,000	16.20%	± 0.4	12.40%	± 0.4
$10,000– $14,999	9.30%	± 0.3	7.80%	± 0.3
$15,000– $24,999	14.10%	± 0.4	14.30%	± 0.5
$25,000–$34,999	11.10%	± 0.3	11.70%	± 0.3
$35,000–$49,999	13.30%	± 0.4	13.70%	± 0.5

TABLE 10.2. Median Family Income, Percent below the Poverty Level, and Number and Percent Less Than 150% of the Poverty Level

	Median family income	% below the poverty level	No. < 150% poverty level	% < 150% of the poverty level
United States	$55,322	22.30%	38,128,868	32.37%
New York State	$60,741	22.30%	2,265,006	31.15%
New York City	$55,191	26.40%	1,100,595	35.24%
The Bronx	$35,302	38.50%	244,595	49.70%

for the target area. The difference between $34,999 and $49,999 is $15,000. The difference between $35,000 and $36,450 is $1,450. Therefore $1,450/$15,000 = X/1.33%. Using this formula we determine that 1.3% has to be added so the percent of families in the Bronx at 150% poverty is 44% + 1.3% or 45.3%. Comparable percentages for families in the state of New York and the United States will also have to be interpolated.

It is also useful to show the contrast between your target area, the larger area, the state, and the United States (see Table 10.2).

American Factfinder also provides information about the educational attainment of your target area. As for the previous criteria, it is useful to contrast educational attainment of your area in comparison to the larger city, the state, and the United States (see Table 10.3).

For the next three criteria, you must obtain information from the specific school or schools that will be served through your project. (The New York State Education Department requires that each public school submit an annual school report. This report contains detailed information on the school. All reports can be accessed through the searchable New York State Education website by name or number of school. The school reports for New York City are also accessible through each individual school website and accessed through **schools. nyc.gov.**) It is likely that many states have centralized data access. One way to determine what might be available for your state is to Google "public school data for X" (insert name of the state that is of interest). I have Googled at least

TABLE 10.3. Educational Attainment

	No high school diploma	High school diploma	BA degree
United States	13.6%	28.0%	29.3%
New York State	13.6%	25.6%	33.7%
New York City	19.9%	24.4%	33.1%
The Bronx	29.3%	27.3%	12.3%

20 states as test cases and have found links to state-level data by specific school in all of them. In each state the data are presented in similar fashion.

These include the selection following selection criteria listed above: *(iii) Dropout rates are high; (iv) College-going rates are low; and (v) Student/counselor ratios are high.* If you are working with several schools, the table should break down the information by school and also provide the comprehensive data across the schools. Each section should have a separate table. The example in Table 10.4 uses student cohort enrollment in one school from 9th to 12th grade/graduation. The overall impact of showing the decreases that occur with a cohort is astounding.

Table 10.5 was created from data collected by the City University of New York (CUNY) over the period 2013–2015. For each year the table shows the number of seniors (and percent of their graduating class) who planned to go to college, and how many of these students (and percent of their graduating class) actually entered a 2-year or 4-year CUNY college. The CUNY system also collects the pass rates on reading, writing, and mathematics entrance examinations so that for each high school the college readiness can be estimated. As the data are comparable between and among schools, it is also possible to generate borough data, county data, or citywide data.

The CUNY system has been tracking these kinds of data for many years as it is useful in determining the impact that system-wide and college-based projects have had on the college readiness of students who might enter CUNY. It is likely that your state university system or education department has similar data on college entrance.

As you cannot expect the external reader to interpret the table exactly as you intend, you need to provide a brief explanation of what you want the reader to note from the data you provide. For greatest impact, you should phrase the explanation using the words of the criteria being illustrated. For example:

> Table 10.5 shows that the college-going rates are extraordinarily low: Of the total seniors (average of 76%) from 2013 to 2015 who indicated that they planned to attend college, an average of 28% attended 2-year colleges and an average of 11% attended 4-year colleges.

TABLE 10.4. Cohort Analysis of Progress to Graduation

Cohort	9th graders	10th graders	11th graders	12th graders	9th graders who graduate
2015–2016	$N = 155$	$N = 117$	$N = 88$	$N = 75$	$N = 75$
		75%	57%	48%	48%
2014–2015	$N = 149$	$N = 119$	$N = 79$	$N = 69$	$N = 69$
		80%	53%	46%	46%

TABLE 10.5. Planned and Actual Postsecondary Enrollment

	N	%	N	%	N	%
Seniors	52	75%	75	77%	98	75%
2-year college	14	26.9%	22	29.3%	27	27.6%
4-year college	6	11.5%	13	17.3%	4	4.1%

CHAPTER SUMMARY

The first and most critical section of the proposal establishes the need for the project. This section is worth 24/100 total points and has several specific items that must be included in a complete response. Each subsection has assigned point values. Several resources are available on the Internet, including the U.S. Census American FactFinder site, where the information needed to complete this section can be found. Local data from schools and community organizations are needed to help complete the evidence required to prove need. Each chart or table presented requires a brief explanation so that the reader can interpret the data correctly. Practice exercises are included after Chapter 18.

Project Goals and Objectives

After establishing the need for your project, you need to present specific and realistic goals for it. This section may include global goals with specific objectives. It is useful to organize the objectives according to the goal each set is designed to accomplish. If the needs/problems are well defined, each goal and associated objectives can be linked to the need it addresses. This makes it easier for readers to see how your project relates to the need it is designed to tackle. Goals describe future expected outcomes and provide programmatic direction. They focus on ends rather than means. Objectives are clear, realistic, specific, measurable, and time-limited. There are two types of objectives: process objective (specify the means to achieve the outcomes) and outcome objectives (address results to be obtained).

As you develop the goals, objectives, and activities, it is useful to note that:

- Goals are related to long-term outcomes;
- Objectives are related to intermediate outcomes; and
- Strategies/activities are related to outputs.

In this section of the proposal, the applicant must present a clear and comprehensive strategy for how the project will be conducted. It must include the procedures and activities that will be utilized or applied in the project. It is essential to indicate what this methodology will accomplish that others haven't.

The examples and explanations below will help you to present a detailed, understandable, and relational overview of the project. I generally use a table that links the needs, objectives, and activities. An example is presented in Table 11.1.

In most RFPs, at least in the past several years, there has been a section entitled "Performance Measures." These are the outcomes that the federal agency releasing the RFP would like to have achieved by the end of the project. For Table 11.2, the performance measures used are from the RFP for the HSI-STEM and Articulation Program (pp. 68–69). This funding is offered by the USDE under the Hispanic-Serving Institutions—Science, Technology, Engineering, or Mathematics and Articulation Programs, CDFA number 84.031C. It is a Title V Strengthening Hispanic-Serving Institutions Program focused on STEM. These are as follows:

1. The percentage change, over the five-year grant period, of the number of Hispanic and low-income full-time STEM field degree-seeking undergraduate students enrolled.
2. The percentage of Hispanic and low-income first-time, full-time STEM field degree-seeking undergraduate students who were in their first year of postsecondary enrollment in the previous year and are enrolled in the current year who remain in a STEM field degree/credential program.
3. The percentage of Hispanic and low-income first-time, full-time degree-seeking undergraduate students enrolled at four-year HSIs graduating within six years of enrollment with a STEM field degree.
4. The percentage of Hispanic and low-income first-time, full-time degree-seeking undergraduate students enrolled at two-year HSIs graduating within three years of enrollment with a STEM field degree/credential.
5. The percentage of Hispanic and low-income students transferring successfully to a four-year institution from a two-year institution and retained in a STEM field major.
6. The number of Hispanic and low-income students participating in grant-funded student support programs or services.
7. The percent of Hispanic and low-income students who participated in grant-supported services or programs who successfully completed gateway courses.
8. The percent of Hispanic and low-income students who participated in grant-supported services or programs in good academic standing.
9. The percent of Hispanic and low-income STEM field major transfer students on track to complete a STEM field degree within three years from their transfer date.
10. The percent of Hispanic and low-income students who participated in grant-supported services or programs and completed a degree or credential.

The reader should see a direct connection/relationship between the needs of the population to be served, the objective you propose, and the activities that

TABLE 11.1. Summary of Objectives, Activities and Evaluative Measures

Performance measure	Objectives	Activities	Evaluative measures
The percentage change, over the 5-year grant period, in the number of Hispanic/low-income full-time STEM-field degree-seeking undergraduate students enrolled.	By [the end of the project period] the number/percent of [identify participants to be served] engaged in the project will increase by 10% as compared to [a group that will not receive support or participate in project activities].	Based on the participants to be served and the needs you have presented (in the needs section), what activities will ensure that you achieve the objective of enrolling/engaging more students?	What aspects of student enrollment or achievement or other parameters will increase as a result of participation in the activities you have identified? What measures will you use to document the change?
The percentage of Hispanic and low-income first-time, full-time STEM-field degree-seeking undergraduate students who enrolled the previous year and remain enrolled in a STEM field degree/credential program.	By [the end of the project period] the number/percent of [identify participants to be served] retained in the project/at the college will increase by 10% as compared to [a group that will not receive support or participate in the project activities].	Based on the participants to be served and the needs you have presented (in the needs section), what activities will ensure that you achieve the objective to retain more students in the project/at the college?	How will you measure student retention in the program/at the college and what measures that might be related to increased retention will you document? What measures will you use to document the student retention?
The percentage of Hispanic and low-income first-time, full-time degree-seeking undergraduate students enrolled at 4-year HSIs graduating within 6 years of enrollment with a STEM field degree.	By [the end of the project period] the number/percentage of [identify participants to be served] graduating within 6 years will increase by 10% as compared to [a group that will not receive support or participate in project activities].	Based on the participants to be served and needs you have presented (in the needs section), what activities will ensure that you achieve the objective to increase the graduation rate so more students graduate within 6 years?	How will you measure student graduation rates and how will you show which activities may have led to the increase?
The percentage of Hispanic and low-income first-time, full-time degree-seeking undergraduate students enrolled at 2-year HSIs graduating within 3 years of enrollment with a STEM field degree/credential.	By [the end of the project period] the percentage of [identify participants to be served] enrolled at 2-year colleges graduating within 3 years of enrollment with [identify program] degree/credential will increase by 10%	Based on the participants to be served and needs you have presented (in the needs section), what activities will ensure that you achieve the objective to increase the graduation rate of students at 2-year colleges so more students graduate within 3 years from entry?	How will you measure student graduation rates and how will you show which activities may have led to the increase?

The percentage of Hispanic and low-income students transferring successfully to a 4-year institution from a 2-year institution and retained in a STEM field major.	By [the end of the project period] the number/percentage of [identify participants to be served] transferring successfully to a 4-year institution from a 2-year institution and retained in a [identify program/major] will increase by 10% as compared to a control group.	How will you measure student graduation rates and how will you show which activities may have led to the increase?
The number of Hispanic/low-income students participating in grant-funded support programs/services; the percentage of Hispanic and low-income students who participated in grant-supported services or programs and successfully completed gateway courses; the percentage of Hispanic and low-income students who participated in grant-supported services or programs in good academic standing.	By [the end of the project period] the number of [population to be served] participating in grant-funded student support programs or services; completing gateway courses in good academic standing, and completing a degree will increase by 10% as compared to a control group.	How will you measure the number and percentage of students who participate in grant programs, complete gateway courses, are in good academic standing, and complete degrees?
The percentage of Hispanic and low-income STEM field major transfer students on track to complete a STEM field degree within 3 years from their transfer date.	By [the end of the project period] the percent of transfer students on track to complete a [designated degree] within 3 years from their transfer date will increase by 10% as compared to a control group.	How will you measure the number and percent of students who complete of a degree by transfer students within three years from their transfer date?

will enable your students to attain the objective. Further, the evaluation measures should relate directly to the objective and be consistent with the information you can glean from the activities you are implementing.

Relationships among Aspects of the Proposal

The reader should see a relationship among the needs, objectives, activities, and evaluation measures.

The objectives presented in Table 11.1 are based on the performance measures included in the RFP. The activities/strategies to be implemented are chosen because they will enable the project to achieve each objective. The evaluative measures enable you to present information on the types of data/information your project will collect to demonstrate that the activities implemented will achieve the objectives.

Table 11.1 presents information from the RFP in table format so that the proposal writer can see how to organize the required information in a way that clearly shows the relationships among required components. Table 11.2 replaces the generic information (from the RFP) with specific information about the proposal to be submitted for funding.

The question now arises: How do you know which activities and strategies will be successful in achieving the objectives you have developed based on the performance measures contained in the RFP? There are several ways of determining this: past experience; research; and high-impact practices. Most important, the activities should relate to the needs you have identified and the objectives they are meant to achieve. In the HSI-STEM RFP guidelines, applicants are asked to provide information on the research that supporting the strategies and activities to be implemented. The results are presented here as Tables 11.3–11.5. A blank template is provided in Form 10. Practice exercises are included after Chapter 18.

Determining the Percentage for Objectives

Proposal objectives must be ambitious (challenging) yet attainable. What percentage change meets these two criteria? You can figure this out by doing the following: gathering local achievement (baseline) data for your target population, accessing research pertaining to the potential impact of your planned activities and interventions for similar populations, and talking to individuals in your organization (perhaps Institutional Research) to get a sense of what is not only possible but achievable.

CHAPTER SUMMARY

The goals and objectives described in this chapter follow from need, discussed in Chapter 10. For some proposals, the objectives are formulated from the selection criteria in the RFP. The institution/organization has to consider the needs, available information about the population to be served, and the desired

TABLE 11.2. Summary of Objectives, Activities, and Evaluative Measures from Actual Funded Proposal

Performance measure	Objectives	Activities	Evaluative measures
The percentage change, over the 5-year grant period, of the number of Hispanic and low-income full-time STEM field degree-seeking undergraduate students enrolled.	By September 2021 the percentage of enrolled Hispanic and low-income full-time STEM field degree-seeking undergraduate students will increase by 10% as compared to a control group.	• Research experience for undergrads (REU) • Winter/summer classes/workshops • Academic support • Guaranteed senior college admission • Long-range academic plan • Intrusive advisement	• Number and percent of participant and nonparticipant undergraduate students in STEM. • Social belonging survey • Attendance at workshops • Enrollment in summer/winter classes
The percentage of Hispanic and low-income first-time, full-time STEM field degree-seeking undergraduate students who were in their first year of postsecondary enrollment in the previous year and are enrolled in the current year who remain in a STEM field degree/credential program	By September 2021 the percentage of retained first-time full-time STEM field degree seeking undergraduate students who were in their first year of postsecondary enrollment in the previous year will increase by 10% as compared to a control group.	• Intrusive advisement • Undergraduate research • Walton et al. and Stephens et al. interventions • Innovative instructional strategies (flipped classroom, use of resources, project-based learning, embedded tutors) academic support in STEM	• GPA • Advisement Sessions • Number of students identified through the Early Warning System • Attendance at workshops • Enrollment in summer/winter classes • Improvement in student perception in STEM.
The percentage of Hispanic and low-income first-time, full-time degree-seeking undergraduate students enrolled at four-year HSIs graduating within 6 years of enrollment with a STEM field degree.	By September 2021 the percentage of Hispanic and low-income first-time, full-time degree-seeking undergraduate students enrolled at 4-year HSIs who graduate within 6 years of enrollment with a STEM field degree will increase by 10%.	• REU • Winter/summer session classes/workshops on the Lehman campus • Long-range academic plan • Academic support intervention • Intrusive advisement • Walton et al. and Stephens et al. interventions	• Credits earned • Time to graduation • No. of/percent advisement sessions • No. of/percent of students identified with EWS • Attendance at workshops • Summer/winter enrollment • Use of academic support • Improvement in student perception in STEM
The percentage of Hispanic and low-income first-time, full-time degree-seeking undergraduate students enrolled at 2-year HSIs graduating within three years of enrollment with a STEM field degree/credential.	By September 2021 the percentage of Hispanic and low-income first-time, full-time degree-seeking undergraduate students enrolled at 2-year HSIs graduating within 3 years of enrollment with a STEM-field degree/credential will increase by 10%.	• REU winter/summer session • Classes/workshops on the Lehman campus • Long-range academic plan • Academic support interventions • Intrusive advisement • Early transfer evaluation • Guaranteed enrollment	• Attendance at workshops • Summer/winter enrollment • No./percent of advisement Sessions • Participation in REU • No./percent of students on track to complete • No./percent of transfers to 4-year college.

(continued)

TABLE 11.2. *(continued)*

Performance measure	Objectives	Activities	Evaluative measures
The percentage of Hispanic and low-income students transferring successfully to a 4-year institution from a 2-year institution and retained in a STEM field major.	By September 2021 the number and percentage of Hispanic and low-income students transferring successfully to a 4-year institution from a 2-year institution and retained in a STEM field major will increase by 10% compared to a control group.	• Undergraduate research • Winter/summer session classes/workshops at Lehman • Long-range academic plan • Academic support interventions • Intrusive advisement	• Number and percent of transfers to 4-year colleges • GPA overall and in STEM-related courses • GPA in gateway courses • Date of transfer evaluation and enrollment at 4-year colleges • Use of academic support
The number of Hispanic and low-income students participating in grant-funded student support programs or services.	By September 2021 the number of Hispanic and low-income students participating in grant-funded student support programs or services, completing gateway courses, in good academic standing and completing a degree will increase by 10% as compared to a control group.	• Intrusive Advisement • Undergraduate Research • Winter/Summer Session—Classes/workshops on the Lehman campus • Long-Range Academic Plan	• Number/percent of students: • Participating in grant programs, completing a Gateway course, in good academic standing, and completing a degree
The percent of Hispanic and low-income STEM field major transfer students on track to complete a STEM field degree within three years from their transfer date.	By September 2021 the percent of Hispanic/low-income STEM major transfer students on track to complete a STEM field degree within 3 years from their transfer date will increase by 10% as compared to a control group.	• Undergraduate research • Winter/summer session Classes/workshops on the Lehman campus • Long-range academic plan • Academic support • Intrusive advisement	• Credits earned • GPA • Time to degree • Number/percent of students on track to complete degree

TABLE 11.3. Summary of Current Research on Student Support Components

Activity	Literature	Summary
Intrusive academic advisement model a. Shared advisement/ retention system b. Financial aid advising	Kolenovic, Z., Linderman, D., & Karp, M. (2013). Improving student outcomes via comprehensive supports. *Community College Review, 41*(4), 271–291. Young-Jones, A. D., Burt, T. D., Dixon, S., & Hawthorne, M. J. (2013). Academic advising: Does it really impact student success? *Quality Assurance In Education: An International Perspective, 21*(1), 7–19. Schwebel, D. C., Walburn, N. C., Klyce, K., & Jerrolds, K. L. (2012). Efficacy of advising outreach on student retention, academic progress and achievement, and frequency of advising contacts: A longitudinal randomized trial. *NACADA Journal, 32*(2), 36–43.	The research articles support the project's use of an intrusive advising model to improve student academic success, retention, and graduation in STEM
Building cultural capital	Walton, G. M., & Cohen, G. L. (2011). A brief social-belonging intervention improves academic and health outcomes of minority students. *Science, 331*(6023), 1447–1451. Stephens, N. M., Hamedani, M. G., & Destin, M. (2014). Closing the social-class achievement gap: A difference-education intervention improves first-generation students' academic performance and all students' college transition. *Psychological Science, 25*(4), 943–953. Walton, G. M., Logel, C., Peach, J., Spencer, S., & Zanna, M. P. (2015). Two brief interventions to mitigate a "chilly" climate transform women's experience, relationships, and achievement in engineering. *Journal of Educational Psychology, 107,* 468–485.	The research cited supports the use of a social belonging intervention, a difference-education intervention, and an affirmation-training intervention to assist students to build cultural capital and to see themselves as members of the higher-education STEM community.
Guaranteed admission with early transfer evaluation and priority registration	Moore, C., & Shulock, N. (2014). *From community college to university: Expectations for California's new transfer degrees*. San Francisco: Public Policy Institute of California. Ott, A. P. (2012). *Transfer credit evaluations at New York State colleges: Comparative case studies of process effectiveness*. Unpublished doctoral dissertation, New York.	The research on early transfer evaluation and priority registration shows a facilitating impact on student enrollment and completion. Information on guaranteed admission is college specific.
Academic support (tutoring, coaching, mentoring, online tutoring, presemester workshops, writing/ literacy in STEM	Reinheimer, D., & McKenzie, K. (2011). The impact of tutoring on the academic succesvs of undeclared students. *Journal of College Reading and Learning, 41*(2), 22–36. Schultheis, S. (2014). *Evaluating an academic support program for urban at-risk college students at a private urban college*. Unpublished doctoral dissertation, Ralph C. Wilson, Jr. School of Education.	Academic support for all students positively impacts grades, retention, and graduation, especially when intrusive advisement assures student compliance with use of resources.

(continued)

TABLE 11.3. *(continued)*

Activity	Literature	Summary
Transitional activities Orientation seminars a. Pretransfer b. Transfer c. Transfer class	Hoffman, A. J., & Wallach, J. (2005). Effects of mentoring on community college students in transition to university. *Community College Enterprise, 11*(1), 67–78. White, K. J. (2012). *Hitting the ground running: The social transition of community college transfer students in an admissions partnership program.* Unpublished master's thesis, Iowa State University, Ames, IA. Lazarowicz, T. A. (2015). *Understanding the transition experience of community college transfer students to a 4-year university: Incorporating Schlossberg's transition theory into higher education.* Unpublished doctoral dissertation, University of Nebraska—Lincoln. Walton, G. M., & Cohen, G. L. (2011). A brief social-belonging intervention improves academic and health outcomes of minority students. *Science, 331*(6023), 1447–1451. Stephens, N. M., Hamedani, M. G., & Destin, M. (2014). Closing the social-class achievement gap: A difference-education intervention improves first-generation students' academic performance and all students' college transition. Psychological *Science, 25*(4), 943–953.	Incorporating high-impact practices to assist transfer students to thrive is reported to be effective. In addition, our project will utilize social-belonging and difference-education initiatives.

outcomes in order to establish reasonable percentages for its objectives. In the grant used as an example, the proposal has to show why the objective is ambitious and attainable: ambitious because of the need that is demonstrated and attainable because of the activities and interventions to be implemented. The best objectives follow the SMART acronym: S = Specific, M = Measurable, A = Attainable, R = Realistic, and T = Time Oriented. In addition, there should be a clear link among needs and objectives, objectives and activities, and objectives, activities, and evaluative measures. In order to receive full credit for the activities you select to realize your objectives, you should provide research citations and evidence. This research is available through the WWC (**https://ies.ed.gov/ncee/wwc**).

TABLE 11.4. Summary of Current Research on Science, Technology, Engineering, and Computer Components

Activity	Literature	Summary
STEM career and professional development with STEM alumni mentors	Tsui, L. (2007). Effective strategies to increase diversity in STEM fields: A review of the research literature. *Journal of Negro Education, 76*(4), 555–581.	Minority students have reported on the critical role that mentors play in their adjustment to college, and progress toward graduate studies and a career (Freeman, 1999; Lee, 1999). Minority students who participated in mentoring programs have demonstrated such positive outcomes as higher grade-point averages, lower attrition, increased self-efficacy, and better-defined academic goals.
Mathematics student academic support a. Enhanced technology in math b. Enhanced academic support	Ni Fhloinn, E., Fitzmaurice, O., Mac an Bhaird, C., & O'Sullivan, C. (2014). Student perception of the impact of mathematics support in higher education. *International Journal of Mathematical Education in Science and Technology, 45*(7), 953–967.	Over 65% of students reported experiencing a positive impact on their approach to, and confidence in, their mathematical ability and grades after intensive mathematics support.
Precalculus project	Hauser, L. A. (2015). Precalculus students' achievement when learning functions: Influences of opportunity to learn and technology from a University of Chicago school mathematics project study. Graduate Theses and Dissertations. Retrieved from *http://scholarcommons.usf.edu/etd/5497.*	The intervention researched in this study had a positive impact on students' understanding of functions related to precalculus.
Summer/winter undergraduate research experiences, intern/externship opportunities	Eagan, M. K., Jr., Hurtado, S., Chang, M. J., Garcia, G. A., Herrera, F. A., & Garibay, J. C. (2013). Making a difference in science education: The impact of undergraduate research programs. *American Educational Research Journal, 50,* 683–713. Allen, D. (2014). Recent research in science teaching and learning. *CBE Life Science Education, 13,* 584–586. Singer, J., & Zimmerman, B. (2012). Evaluating a summer undergraduate research program: Measuring student outcomes and program impact. *Council on Undergraduate Research Quarterly, 32*(3), 40–47. Retrieved from *www.cur.org/download.aspx?id=2842.* Robnett, R. D., Chemer, M., & Zurbriggen, E. (2015). Longitudinal associations among undergraduates' research experience, self-efficacy, and identity. *Journal of Research in Science Teaching, 52*(6), 847–867.	The incorporation of a research experience for undergraduates is well supported as a high-impact practice that increases enrollment and retention in STEM majors and also increases the graduation rates, especially for Hispanic and low-income students.

TABLE 11.5. Summary of Current Research on Curriculum Revision Components

Activity	Literature	Summary
Develop AS in liberal arts and sciences for transfer		
Comprehensive STEM agreement leveraging 70-credit transfer policy	For students enrolled in STEM AA/AS programs, this change of policy allows students to successfully graduate with the AA/AS degree without needing to place in calculus. Students who place in college algebra, statistics, or precalculus will be able to complete degree requirements without fearing loss of credit. The implementation of this policy will allow students to maximize credits accepted in transfer and fully utilize financial aid, and ultimately it will positively impact degree completion.	Research leading up to the adoption of this policy revealed that the extra credits would have a positive impact on student success after transfer.
Incorporate active learning strategies and peer mentors	Freeman, S., Eddy, S., McDonough, M., Smith, M., Okoroafor, N., Jordt, H., et al. (2014). Active learning increases performance in science, engineering and mathematics. *Proceedings of the National Academy of Science of the USA, 111*(23), 8319–8320.	This meta-analysis concludes that active learning strategies positively impact student understanding and learning in STEM.

CHAPTER 12

Plan of Operation

- What is a Plan of Operation?
- What are the subsections of the Plan of Operation section for a proposal?
- Do the sections here apply to all grants even if not specifically shown in the RFP?

- What tables and charts do I need to include?
- What is an organizational chart?
- How can I easily create organizational charts?

The Plan of Operation section contains several important subsections as shown below. This section is required for TRIO programs (Talent Search, Upward Bound, Student Support Services, and the McNair Scholars Program) but is useful to guide your thinking and planning for other competitions. Although these headings are specific for TRIO grants, the elements provide an overview of what might be included in any proposal. You should think of the Plan of Operation as a cookbook or procedures manual for how your project will be conducted. You need to be precise and concise. Often the Plan of Operation section of your proposal can be used as an operations manual that all leaders and staff for the project can use to guide their actions and activities. Practice exercises are located after Chapter 18.

(c) Plan of operation (30 points). The Secretary evaluates the quality of the applicant's plan of operation on the basis of the following:

(1) (3 points) The plan to inform the institutional community (students, faculty, and staff) of the goals, objectives, and services of the project and the eligibility requirements for participation in the project.

(2) (3 points) The plan to identify, select, and retain project participants with academic need.

(3) (4 points) The plan for assessing each individual participant's need for specific services and monitoring his or her academic progress at the institution to ensure satisfactory academic progress.

(4) (10 points) The plan to provide services that address the goals and objectives of the project.

(5) (10 points) The applicant's plan to ensure proper and efficient administration of the project, including the organizational placement of the project; the time commitment of key project staff; the specific plans for financial management, student records management, and personnel management; and, where appropriate, its plan for coordination with other programs for disadvantaged students.

(a) Plan of Operation. The Secretary determines the quality of the applicant's plan of operation on the basis of the following.

(1) (3 points) The plan to inform the institutional community (students, faculty, and staff) of the goals, objectives, and services of the project and the eligibility requirements for participation in the project.

The reader will evaluate your proposal on how you will let college personnel and staff and participating schools and community organizations know about the project. For faculty and staff at your institution it might take the form of an e-mail blast; an announcement on the college website; presentations at faculty meetings; meetings with involved departments/schools; and meetings with faculty to be engaged in delivering services.

It is also critical that the local community, parents and families, local service organizations, school districts, and local schools are informed about the project, eligibility, enrollment, activities, and contacts. Methods might include newspaper articles, presentations at parent meetings, announcements in school and other bulletins, presentations at teacher and parent meetings at local schools, and letters home to parents/guardians in the various languages of the community.

You should indicate, in the proposal, what key information you will share with your constituencies, including a brief paragraph that highlights the roles and contributions expected from inside and outside your organization. In section 5 of the Plan of Operation you will indicate how various offices within your institution, participating schools/organizations, and community members will contribute to the project. You might wish to indicate that these promised offerings will be highlighted in your communication to partners.

> **Informing Constituencies**
>
> You should consider including a paragraph outlining the information you will present to organizational staff and community organizations.

In programs in which the institution is working with outside agencies/schools or other institutions, a cooperative agreement or memorandum of understanding (MOU) specifying the responsibilities of each partner will demonstrate to reviewers that partners have engaged in planning and discussions to assure a successful collaboration. (A sample MOU is included in Appendix D.) The agreement might include information about assistance in identifying students, providing student information, space for program activities at the school, collaboration with school staff, support by teachers and principals, attendance at parent and teacher meetings, circulation of program information flyers, and a school site office for program staff. In addition, the agreement will detail what the institution is expected to provide: space at the college, supplies, books and materials, staff for summer and academic year classes/workshops, maintenance of a student database, confidentiality for students, tutoring services as needed, college access activities, and opportunity for qualified students to enroll in tuition-waived college credit courses.

(2) (3 points) The plan to identify, select, and retain project participants with academic need.

In this section, the proposal should use the language of the RFP pertaining to criteria presented for participants and for the assurances the institution must provide regarding the participants.

Many RFPs stipulate eligibility criteria for participation. This is especially true for TRIO, HSI, HBCU, and Title V programs of the United States Department of Education and increasingly the case for NSF, USDA, and other funding agencies that have created set-aside programs for underrepresented groups. In the case where eligibility criteria are provided, it is essential that you provide clear information on how you will identify and select participants according to the RFP. Language from TRIO Upward Bound, for example, states that:

> **Eligibility Criteria**
>
> Increasingly RFPs stipulate eligibility requirements for participants. You need to clearly define your requirements so that they match what is required and indicate how you will verify eligibility.

§ 645.3 Who is eligible to participate in an Upward Bound project?

An individual is eligible to participate in a Regular, Veterans, or a Math and Science Upward Bound project if the individual meets all of the following requirements:

(a)

(1) Is a citizen or national of the United States.

(2) Is a permanent resident of the United States.

(3) Is in the United States for other than a temporary purpose and provides evidence from the Immigration and Naturalization Service of his or her intent to become a permanent resident.

(4) Is a permanent resident of Guam, the Northern Mariana Islands, or the Trust Territory of the Pacific Islands.

(5) Is a resident of the Freely Associated States—the Federated States of Micronesia, the Republic of the Marshall Islands, or the Republic of Palau.

(b) Is—

    (1) A potential first-generation college student;

    (2) A low-income individual; or

    (3) An individual who has a high risk for academic failure.

(c) Has a need for academic support, as determined by the grantee, in order to pursue successfully a program of education beyond high school.

(d) At the time of initial selection, has completed the 8th grade and is at least 13 years old but not older than 19, although the Secretary may waive the age requirement if the applicant demonstrates that the limitation would defeat the purposes of the Upward Bound program. However, a veteran as defined in §645.6, regardless of age, is eligible to participate in an Upward Bound project if he or she satisfies the eligibility requirements in paragraphs (a), (b), and (c) of this section.

The RFP goes on to specify the percentages of low-income and potential first-generation students comprising the total enrollment. These are:

§ 645.21 What assurances must an applicant include in an application?

(a) An applicant for a Regular Upward Bound award must assure the Secretary that—

    (1) Not less than two-thirds of the project's participants will be low-income individuals who are potential first-generation college students;

    (2) The remaining participants will be low-income individuals, potential first-generation college students, or individuals who have a high risk for academic failure;

    (3) No student will be denied participation in a project because the student would enter the project after the 9th grade; and

    (4) The project will collaborate with other Federal TRIO projects, GEAR UP projects, or programs serving similar populations that are serving the same target schools or target area in order to minimize the duplication of services and promote collaborations so that more students can be served.

(3) (4 points) The plan for assessing each individual participant's need for specific services and monitoring his or her academic progress at the institution to ensure satisfactory academic progress.

All program implementation proposals are designed around the needs of the projected participants. It is crucial, especially in TRIO grants and those proposing services in HSI, HBCU, Title V set-asides, and other RFPs targeting specific underrepresented populations, that information on assessing needs and monitoring the progress of participants be specifically detailed in the proposal.

As noted in previous sections, this information can be presented in paragraph form or, if applicable, can be in a single-spaced table (if permitted by the RFP formatting).

Assessments, which may also be used as part of the evaluation process, can include academic measures such as standardized test scores, course grades, attendance, behavior, class participation, state test scores, grade-point average, required admissions essay, and credits attempted versus credits earned. Noncognitive measures, while more difficult to assess, would make your proposal stand out. They include academic skills, achievement, motivation, self-management, and social support (**www.studentachievement.org**).

> ***Noncognitive Skills***
>
> **These include confidence, curiosity, persistence, organization, discipline, motivation, creativity, adaptability, integrity, trust, ethics, and initiative.**

(4) (10 points) The plan to provide services that address the goals and objectives of the project.

It is likely that the readers will not know what processes/procedures are inherent in implementation of each of the activities, and you should not assume that they understand how you will define them. It is useful to describe each of the activities in terms of how it will be implemented in the project. This can be done in narrative form (as paragraphs); if the formatting rules allow single spacing of tables and charts, then a table would be preferable. Note that you must read the formatting section of the RFP very carefully as different RFPs may have different formatting regulations. There is usually a specific section that specifies page size, typeface, margins, line spacing, number of pages permitted, and formatting of tables, figures, and charts. In some cases, tables and charts can be single spaced; recently this has changed to all text, charts, tables, and headings must be double spaced.

Table 12.1 provides examples of activities and descriptions. It also follows the logic model somewhat and includes additional information which demonstrates that the planning has been thorough and that the activities are related to the logic model (Chapter 9). It is critical that all tables containing similar information be consistent. The evaluation measures in one table should not be different from the evaluation measures in another table. For that reason I again recommend having a Master Table with all of the information needed in all tables and editing out the columns or information you do not need for each table in the proposal. In the evaluation section, for example, you will need the objectives and the performance measures, so you would copy the Master Table and delete all columns you do not need for this section. Table 12.1 was excerpted from the Master Table by deleting all but the Activity, Description, Output, Outcomes, Measures, and Leader columns. A blank template is provided in Form 11.

TABLE 12.1. HSI-STEM Activities, Description, Output, Outcomes, Measures, and Leader (Innovative Student Services for College Success)

Target group: Low-income, first-generation-college Hispanic students at 2- and 4-year colleges as first-time freshmen and as transfers

Goal: Increase number of transfers and completion of associate of arts, associate of science, and baccalaureate degrees in STEM

Activities	Description	Output	Outcomes	Measures	Leader
Intrusive academic advisement model a. Shared advisement/ retention system b. Financial aid advising	Proactive advisement with high degree of contact a. Shared tool for advisement and retention b. Dedicated financial aid adviser(s) at both college levels; financial planning seminars.	Monitor student progress, share case notes, provide follow-up reports • On-time financial aid and FAFSA filing • Track financial aid	a. Improved academic achievement; higher retention; seamless transition; continuation of student advisement record b. Early application, maximize aid eligibility	• GPA • Retention rate • Students served are successful	Project director; academic advisement director; technical director; financial aid directors
Guaranteed admission with priority registration Create cohort group	Participants agree to fulfill requirements (degree, GPA, proficiency, general education, and STEM courses) and are guaranteed admission with early registration	Students know what must be accomplished for admission to Senior College • Process seamless • Students sign admission agreement	Successful transition to senior college with degree in 2–3 years; transfer evaluation done early; students get classes they need and make good progress; admission/completion	• No./percent of students in cohort enrolling at Lehman • No. of credits taken • Adherence to requirements	Admission directors at the participating colleges
Academic support (tutoring, coaching, mentoring, online tutoring,	Academic tutoring/coaching offered to freshmen/sophomores; mentoring for junior/senior; two	• Tutoring available immediately • Academic coaches available spring 2017 and thereafter.	• Student understanding • Improved attendance • Surveys	• Measures of self-efficacy, course grades, GPA	STEM academic support coordinators

presemester workshops, writing/literacy in stem, weekend review sessions)	or more appointments per week with academic coach; workshops support students' writing in science; review sessions for STEM courses	• Workshops planned in fall 2017–spring 2018 and offered in the summer after year 2	• Self-efficacy	• Improved grades, retention, graduation rates • Survey • Improved writing	
Orientation Incoming freshmen, community/senior colleges	Precollege orientation for freshmen Completion of closing the achievement gap protocol	Students have pre-knowledge of tools, policies, and procedures to succeed in college	Successful college entry; improved self-perception; increase in cultural capital for college	• Retention • GPA • Survey results • Sense of belonging	Admissions advisers Academic advisers
Transitional orientation for community college a. Pretransfer b. Transfer c. Transfer class	a. Facilitate pretransfer seminar (at the community college) to prepare STEM students b. Address the following issues: campus culture; resources for success; expectations; transfer courses; building connections c. Elective course for STEM transfer students to foster connection/engagement for retention	Students have pre-knowledge of tools, policies, and procedures at Senior College; students prepared to navigate Senior College resources and campus Students know Lehman infrastructure, student support options, office and department locations	• Successful transition to Lehman • Offices for assistance • Location of departments • Familiar with campus culture • Know Lehman students as members of project cohort	• Transfer rates into science majors • Survey results • Retention • GPA • Survey results • Sense of belonging	Admissions codirectors Admissions advisers Academic advisers

(5) (10 points) The applicant's plan to ensure proper and efficient administration of the project, including the organizational placement of the project; the time commitment of key project staff; the specific plans for financial management, student records management, and personnel management; and, where appropriate, its plan for coordination with other programs for disadvantaged students.

This section includes many items, and the writer would be wise to use subheadings for each aspect so that the reader can easily determine that all of the areas have been addressed. I have organized the material below in the same order, using subheadings as stated in the criteria.

Organizational Placement of the Project

The reader will evaluate and assign a point value to the description of where you will locate the project within your organization. I use software to create an easily understandable figure that shows the reporting structure for the project. I use SmartDraw but there are other programs that will do the same thing. Before discovering SmartDraw I used Excel but found it very tedious, especially when having to edit the figure. Other programs that can be used to create organizational charts are Lucidchart, OrgPlus, and Organimi. Microsoft Office also states that Word and PowerPoint can be used to create such charts.

Figure 12.1 presents the management chart showing positions for the HSI-STEM grant.

The positions included in Figure 12.1 will also be included in the next section, Time Commitment of Key Project Staff. It is important that all of the positions described in the organizational chart be included in that section and that information on reporting lines be the same as pictured in the figure. Remember that an observant reader might compare the organizational chart with the Roles and Responsibilities Table.

The proposal writer should not assume that the external reader will be familiar with your institution (or institutions similar to yours) and so should include a descriptive paragraph after the organizational figure explaining the reporting structure, how much autonomy the committees have, how reporting is managed to be sure that there is a cohesive approach to the project, and what the abbreviations in some of the cells mean. It might be useful to have a brief role and responsibility chart here as a summary for the reader.

Figure 12.1 is complex because there are three different colleges collaborating on the project and it was necessary to show how representatives from each college will work together to implement the program. A simpler organizational chart for a project from one institution is shown in Figure 12.2.

The text that would go with the organizational Figure 12.1 might read as follows:

> Figure 12.1 indicates the reporting/organizational structure for the project. There are three institutions collaborating on this program and in all cases responsible teams

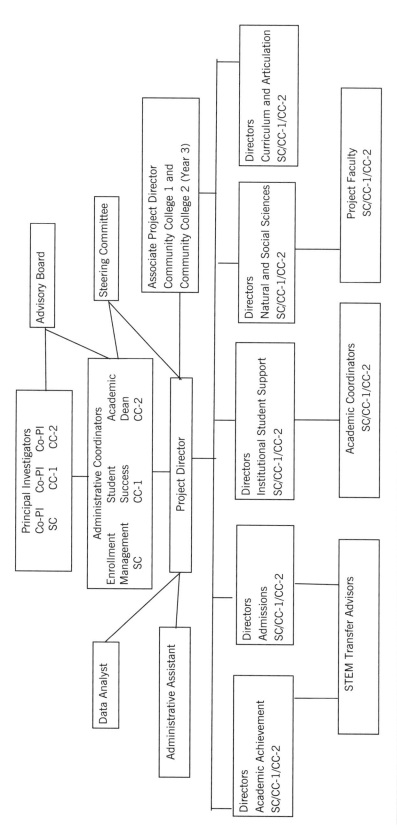

FIGURE 12.1. Complex organizational chart for multi-institution collaboration. *Note:* SC = senior college; CC-1 = community college 1; CC-2 = community college 2.

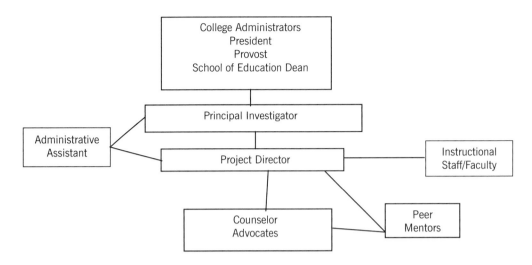

FIGURE 12.2. Simple organizational chart for a single organization.

are comprised of representatives of each of the institutions: one is a 4-year college and the other two are 2-year colleges. The 4-year college serves as the fiscal agent. The PI [principal investigator] team includes a senior administrator from each of the institutions, as does the administrative team and the teams that guide decision making regarding academic advisement, admissions, student support, natural and social sciences content, and curriculum and articulation. The advisory board works with the PI team and the administrative coordinators to provide strategic advice on various aspects of the project. The steering committee provides continuous support, guidance, and oversight to the project director and other individuals involved in the day-to-day implementation of the project. The data analyst works with the administrative team and through them with the project director to assure that the data collection and analysis reflects the evaluation process approved in the proposal. The administrative assistant works with the project director to assure that the project activities run smoothly and that deadlines are met. Finally, the transfer advisers, academic coordinators, and faculty report to the appropriate team of directors from each institution with regular intra and interinstitutional meetings.

As can be noted in Figure 12.2, the organizational chart is much simpler with direct lines from college administration to the PI and the PI to the project director. The project director oversees the counselor advocates and the peer mentors/tutors. The administrative assistant works with both the PI and the PD on day-to-day aspects of the project.

Time Commitment of Key Project Staff

It is useful here to present a table detailing the qualifications, responsibilities, and time commitments of the key personnel in the project. The information on the key individuals in your organization who will oversee the project can be presented in short paragraphs detailing their qualifications, past responsibilities, and successes. Detail on specific responsibilities of all key personnel as well as their time commitment is important. This includes qualifications for all positions you will fill for the project. Those shown in the organizational management figure include Project Director, Associate Project Director, Administrative Assistant, STEM Transfer Advisors, Academic Coordinators, and Project Faculty. The résumés of all known key personnel should be included in an appendix. The use of a table here is also helpful. Table 12.2, from the funded project used as an example, illustrates how the information on duties and time commitments can be presented.

Timeline for Project

Use of a timeline or chart to demonstrate how the activities and accomplishments of your project will be sequenced indicates that you have thought about and considered when events should occur and how long they will take (see Table 12.3). Also important to include is who will be responsible for completion of the activities and who will be responsible for seeing that the timelines are followed. The timeline demonstrates that the applicant has "guideposts" for when specific achievements should take place. The milestones can be bullet points and, if possible, contain specific months. If the timeline column is narrow, additional dates are not necessary.

A lack of time-specific milestones, and/or lack of staff responsible for achieving those milestones, implies a lax system. It suggests the applicant has not thought about implementing the project or is not prepared to do so.

Financial Management

The proposal should provide specific information about fiscal responsibility for the project. Usually it is the project director, assisted by an administrator, who is responsible for project financial management. When there is a PI, he or she has final responsibility for fiscal matters. Depending on your system of managing grant awards, the administrator might want to independently track program expenses so that fiscal reports can be checked for accuracy. Depending on how your grant funds are managed, your administrator may want to set up and maintain a tracking system so that the income and expenses can be reviewed regularly against centralized reports from the fiscal management organization.

If students will be given stipends, an explanation for when and how stipends are disbursed should include the criteria for receipt of stipends during the academic year and during the summer. This explanation should include *amounts, attendance criteria, minimum participation rules, and who will issue the checks.* If your institution has a fiscal agent, then information about that person should be

TABLE 12.2. Project Personnel Time Commitment, Qualifications, and Responsibilities

Title	% Time	Qualifications	Responsibilities
Principal Investigator	3% (in-kind)	Key positions in each participating organization with the authority to recommend/oversee needed changes	• Provide institutional support for the project; facilitate adoption of curricular changes; meet with project at least two times a year
Administrative Coordinators	7% (in-kind)	Key positions in each participating college; have oversight for the areas of admissions, curriculum, career counseling, strategic planning	• Project budget oversight; ensure project activities adhere to specifications in the budget; • Work toward institutionalization; meet with steering/advisory committee
Project Director	100%	• Master's or doctorate degree in appropriate area of specialization; 5 years academic advising experience particularly in working with Hispanic and low-income students; supervisory experience in an office setting; excellent communication skills • Experience in higher education or related area • Community college experience preferred	• Ensure realization of objectives through close coordination with administrative coordinators/steering committee • Collaborate with Office of Institutional Research to establish data collection procedures/ensure that appropriate/accurate data are collected • Communicate concerning activities, potential problems, and performance measures • Comply with federal regulations, rules, and procedures regarding administration of the grant; ensure that modifications to the plan are made with appropriate approvals
Associate Director	100%	• Master's or doctorate degree in an appropriate area of specialization (STEM areas preferred). ≥3 years' academic advising experience, particularly in working with Hispanic and low-income students Supervisory experience in an office setting; Excellent communication skills; • Experience in higher education or related area; • Community college experience preferred	• Serve as liaison to community colleges • Work with Lehman transfer center • Coordinate activities with administrative coordinators and steering committee • Meet weekly with project director • Collaborate with the Offices of Institutional Research at the community colleges to establish data collection procedures and ensure that appropriate and accurate data are collected • Work closely with academic advisers at the community college campus • Assist in recruiting students at the community colleges
Data Analyst and Administrative Assistant	50% Yr 1 100% Yrs 2–5	• 4 years' experience with data collection, statistical evaluation, large data sets, and data mining; familiar with a variety of data packages; experience with building or designing data collection screens; familiar with higher education data requirements/conventions	• Build/design data input/collection screens with steering committee and evaluator; Import, clean, transform, validate and model data for the purpose of decision making • Present data in charts, graphs, tables, design/develop relational databases for collecting data • Improve data quality and present conclusions gained from analyzing data using statistical tools • Perform administrative assistant duties

(continued)

TABLE 12.2. *(continued)*

Title	% Time	Qualifications	Responsibilities
Academic Advisers (2): one at CC-1/CC-2 one at SC	100%	• Master's degree in an appropriate area of specialization • 2 years' academic advising experience, particularly in working with at-risk students • Excellent communication skills • Computer skills to access student information database, clear registration holds, and prepare appropriate reports • Community college experience preferred	• The adviser, cross-trained in advisement, admissions and financial aid policies, will be located at CC-1 (and adding CC-2 in year 3) to meet with cohort and individual students on a regular basis • Advise students on academic policies, degree requirements, admissions process and financial aid to ensure they stay on track and are successful in completing their degree and for community college students ready to transfer
Part-time STEM Career advisor	50%	• Bachelor's degree in psychology, social work, counseling, student services or related area; master's degree preferred 4 years' counseling experience required • Counseling experience in institution of higher education preferred • Excellent verbal, writing, interpersonal, and organizational skills • Community college experience a plus • Ability to function well in an energetic and creative team environment • Knowledge of web-based career systems, career-building technologies and administrative software essential • Committed to serving a diverse, urban student population	• Guide students in their career journey through coaching, career exploration, career development workshops, mentoring, internships, and relevant career activities that will broaden students' perspective and experience in STEM • Develop/implement career workshops, career identification, career exploration tools for work with students in groups and individually
STEM Academic Support Coordinator in the Institutional Student Support Programs	40%	• Bachelor's degree required • Master's degree in STEM or related area preferred; experience in higher education, tutoring/academic support, and teaching, as well as knowledge of STEM pedagogy and academic support (tutoring, supplemental instruction, peer-led team learning) and student engagement strategies; ability to work collaboratively; proven record of excellent interpersonal/organizational, writing/communication skills required	• Coordinator hires/trains/supervises tutors and other academic support personnel; oversees design of services/support materials for STEM students; collaborates with STEM faculty/staff across the college and at grant partner institutions to enhance classroom/out of classroom support services to increase retention in STEM. Works with ISSP staff to evaluate and assess STEM academic support initiatives, collects data on program services, creates reports to meet grant reporting requirements, and contributes to reports. Assists the ISSP director and STEM grant PI with other functions as needed to support STEM education at the college.
Academic coaches, mentors, personal peer mentors	10 hours/ week	• Upper-division or master's students with high grades in STEM courses; excellent understanding of concepts in STEM fields; good communication skills; able to explain difficult concepts and provide real-world examples; good rapport with other students; able to teach rather then tell	• Academic coaches will focus on helping small groups of students to develop highly effective habits that can range from strategic thinking to problem solving, to oral communication/presentation skills; work with faculty and staff to foster relationships and cross-campus support for their STEM cohort; monitor student progress for group members.

Note. ALAS = Associate degree in Liberal Arts and Sciences; CC-1 = community college 1; CC-2 = community college 2; ISSP = Integrated Student Support Program; SC = senior college.

TABLE 12.3. Project Timeline

Timeline	Milestones	Responsible individual
Summer 2016	Once the grant is submitted; the PIs and the administrative coordinators will meet with the college directors (SC and CC-1) participating in oversight of project services to assure that the management and reporting paths and responsibilities are clear.	Administrative coordinators
October 2016 to December 2016	• Search processes initiated • Hiring complete for project director, administrative assistant, and data analyst • Initial steering committee (monthly) • Hiring complete for associate project director • Review of freshmen at SC and CC-1 to identify participants • Recruitment of undergraduates • Preliminary screening/preassessment • Planning of winter undergraduate courses/research experiences • Identify/train student tutors, mentors, coaches • Advisory committee meeting (web based) • Identify STEM programs at CC-1 for comprehensive articulation • Complete guaranteed admission agreement with CC-1 • Recruit students for guaranteed admission	Administrative coordinators Steering committee Evaluators Academic adviser
January 2017	• Offer initial winter session Research Experience for Undergraduates (REU) • Offer winter session courses in Math • Conduct preliminary screening and preassessments as proposed in evaluation plan • Continue to identify/recruit undergrads • Hiring completed for STEM advisers for SC/CC-1 • Create electronic student group comprised of participants • Continue to identify/train student tutors, mentors, coaches	Project director Faculty instructors Registrar Staff leaders Data analyst
February 2017 to May 2017	• Continue to identify/recruit students • Continue to identify/train tutors, mentors, coaches, peer mentors • Hiring completed for STEM Career Advisor • Outreach to incoming students • Hiring completed for ISSP Coordinator of STEM Academic Services • Steering committee meets monthly • Design teams continue project director sessions • Design summer REU • Project events for students • Recruit students to participate in summer REU • Form working group to develop AS degree in liberal arts and sciences • Discuss STEM articulation agreement for submission • Complete five additional articulation agreements with CC-1	Project director Campuses director Steering committee Faculty Academic advisers
June 2017 to August 2017	• Summer REU for SC and CC-1 HSI-STEM students • Summer courses for math and gateway sciences • Advisory committee meeting (in person)	Project director Faculty instructors

(continued)

TABLE 12.3. *(continued)*

Timeline	Milestones	Responsible individual
September 2017 to December 2017	• Begin planning with CC-2 for implementation in September 2018 • Continue to identify and recruit undergraduates • Continue to identify and train student tutors, mentors, coaches, personal peer mentors • Hiring completed for STEM career adviser • Outreach to incoming students • Hiring completed for ISSP Coordinator of STEM Academic Services • Steering committee meetings (monthly) • Design summer undergraduate research experience • Project events for students/faculty at SC and CC-1 • Recruit SC and CC-1 STEM students to participate in winter REU • Submit ASLAS to CC-1 governance • Submit five articulation agreements	Administrative coordinators Project director Campus director Advisers Academic support personnel Faculty instructors Registrar Staff leaders Data analyst
January 2018	• Advisory committee meeting (web based) • Winter REU activities • Winter courses as needed	Administrative coordinators Project director Faculty instructors Advisers
February 2018 to May 2018	• Orientation, transfer evaluation, and registration for CC-1 students entering SC • Final implementation planning with CC-2 administrators and personnel for September 2018 • Continue to identify and recruit undergraduates • Continue to Identify and train student tutors, mentors, coaches • Hiring completed for STEM Career Advisor • Outreach to incoming students • Hiring completed for ISSP Coordinator of STEM Academic Services • Steering committee meetings (monthly) • Design teams continue Professional Development Opportunities • Design summer undergraduate research experience • Project events for students/faculty at SC and CC-1 • Recruit SC and CC-1 STEM students for summer research	Administrative coordinators Project director Campus director advisers Academic support personnel Faculty instructors Registrar Staff leaders Data analyst
June 2018 to August 2018	• Summer REU for SC and CC-1 HSI-STEM students • Summer courses for math and gateway sciences • Advisory committee meeting (in person) • Welcoming reception for CC-1 students entering SC	Project director Faculty instructors Advisers
September 2018 to December 2018	• CC-2 STEM student participants complete orientation and pre-program evaluations • STEM Advisor splits time between CC-1/CC-2 • Begin recruiting for ASLAS • Conduct review of articulation agreements • Identify STEM programs for comprehensive articulation agreement with CC-2 • Complete guaranteed admission agreement with CC-2	Administrative coordinators Project director Campus director Advisers Academic support personnel Faculty instructors Staff leaders Data analyst
January 2019	• Advisory committee meeting (web based) • Winter REU activities (SC, CC-1, CC-2) • Winter courses as needed (SC, CC-1, CC-2)	Administrative coordinators Project director Faculty instructors Advisers
February 2019 to August 2021	• Activities and meetings continue as in previous years with addition of CC-2 personnel and students • Complete five STEM articulation agreements with CC-2 • Implement guaranteed admission agreement with CC-2	Program staff as previously identified

Note. ALAS = Associate degree in Liberal Arts and Sciences; CC-1 = community college 1; CC-2 = community college 2; ISSP = Integrated Student Support Program; SC = senior college.

included here as well as the role assumed with reference to tracking and reporting on spending, and you should state the project will have sound fiscal management and comply with standard accounting principles.

Fiscal Agent

The fiscal agent oversees grant funds and assures that funds are spent in accordance with federal, state or foundation regulations. The fiscal agent tracks expenditures, provides fiduciary oversight, financial management, and other administrative services. Most educational institutions have sponsored program or grants offices that act as fiscal agents for grants. University systems may have centralized fiscal agents. For example, the City University of New York has the Research Foundation of CUNY as the fiscal agent for all federal and state grants. Individual colleges may have a foundation or institutional advancement office to oversee corporate or foundation funding. In the case of cooperative grants between or among institutions one must be the lead institution and take the role of fiscal agent.

Student Records Management

Who will maintain the student records and where will they be stored? Who will have access? Will a software program such as Blumen, Access, or Excel be used to keep track of enrollment, participation, attendance, grades, credits earned, courses taken, and standardized tests? How will data be backed up and secured? How will reports to principals, counselors, teachers, and parents be prepared and what will they contain? What will physical student files contain? (Possible examples include eligibility data; student intake information; signed parental permission forms for trips and attendance at Saturday and summer programs; individualized attendance record; needs assessment data; educational plan; citywide test scores; standardized test scores; regents examination scores; progress reports; academic transcripts; advising reports; student activities transcripts; copies of recommendations and applications for college; director's, coordinator's, teachers', counselors', and advisers' notes; writing samples from selected courses; and tracking information regularly printed from the database.) Will the information be scanned and placed in electronic files and/or will paper copies be stored?

Personnel Management

The proposal should provide detailed information on your institution's hiring process and the specific guidelines to be used. Where will announcements be posted? How will you assure that personnel will reflect the population to be served by the project? Is your institution an Equal Opportunity Employer (EOE) and do you adhere to Americans with Disabilities Act (ADA) requirements? You need to check that *actual* institutional EOE policies and compliance with the ADA and the Civil Rights Act *should*—but not always—already be codified by the applicant agency. If your organization has these policies, there will be a statement that you should quote in this section of your proposal. A sample statement might read as follows:

It is the policy of [name of organization] to recruit, employ, retain, promote, and provide benefits to employees and to admit and provide services for students without regard to race, color, national or ethnic origin, religion, age, sex, sexual orientation, gender identity, marital status, disability, genetic predisposition or carrier status, alienage, citizenship, military or veteran status, or status as a victim of domestic violence.

You should keep copies of these policies on hand to share or inform your work. If you find that your agency does not have these policies, you should not describe them in your proposal.

Who will oversee personnel and who will be responsible for supervising, locating, and providing professional development opportunities to program staff? In describing the reporting relationships you should refer back to the organizational chart or figure that you have presented and be sure that the information presented there is consistent with your description in this part of the Plan of Operation. Will professional development opportunities be offered? How will personnel be assessed and evaluated? How and how often will student progress be reviewed and by whom? Who will have access to the database and how will it be protected? Who will be able to update student information, grades, and attendance in the program database? How will the relationship with students, parents, and others be maintained?

College/Community Resources

Most funders and regulations in the Education Department General Administrative Regulations specify that grants must be used to supplement, not supplant. The funds received may not be used to shore up budget shortfalls or to provide services that are covered by the institutional budget. Therefore, the RFP usually includes a request for how currently available institutional resources and personnel might/will be used to realize the goals and objectives of the project. You

> **Supplement, not Supplant**
>
> In practice, the prohibition against supplanting under any grant award means that recipients may not use those funds to pay for services that, in the absence of external funds, would be provided by other federal, state, or local funds.

should identify the departments of the college that offer services to the participants you propose to serve and ask them if they might offer special workshops/events that provide specific information for project participants. These areas might include financial aid, career services, library workshops, community service, support services, and academic advisement and departments. There may also be college events that take place on a regular basis that participants might be specifically invited to attend as a group and then participate in follow-up discussion.

It is also likely that your college or the schools you work with have other projects offering opportunities for underrepresented students and/or their parents or that the other projects offer different and useful services in which your students can participate. Some colleges have outreach or community programs that offer workshops and courses for adult learners/community members. Arrangements for program participant parents or siblings to participate would deepen connections between the participants' families and the college. The MOU (see Appendix D) completed by each school/partner in the project will indicate its participation and contribution.

In order to provide information on the contributions of your organization/ institution, a table such as Table 12.4 would detail the participation of people and offices within your institution and its value.

Tracking Graduates

As noted in the performance measures presented in Chapter 11, the objectives and outcomes include maintaining information about the impact of the program on participants. A successful follow-up plan requires preplanning on how to engage students as members of a community and to establish strong

TABLE 12.4. Summary of College Contributions

Office/personnel	Activity/service	Time schedule	Contrib/yr
Financial Aid Office Counselor	Financial aid workshops for parents and participants	Once each semester of each project year	$2,000
Career Services Director	Provide access to career services computers and programming	After school as scheduled for 5–10 students per week	$8,000
College Relations Director	Preparation/dissemination of news releases	Monthly	$3,000
Admissions Office	Provide admissions workshops for 11th-/12th-grade students.	Twice each semester of each project year	$4,000
Multilingual Journalism	Translations of flyers, letters, brochures	As needed	$2,000
Information Technology Center	Use of computers on Saturdays and in the summer program	20 Saturdays/year and 30 days in summer	$12,000
College Now	PSAT/SAT workshops; regents preparation; college credit cohort courses; regularly scheduled college courses.	School year: after school and on Saturdays; two sections of each every semester.	$15,000
Lehman College	Office space, furniture, Internet connection, phone service, e-mail service	Duration of project— amount in excess of indirect costs	$10,000
Academic Support	Math lab, academic center, gymnasium	Tutoring, recreational activities during the school year and on Saturdays.	$5,000
Division of Education (provided by school/college technology funding)	Computer mobile carts, smart boards, computerized science probes	In-school activities will use the equipment/resources on Saturdays and during the summer.	$40,000

connections among students and between students and program staff. In many cases the college major department and the project personnel who have the closest relationship with the student are in the best position to maintain contact over time. These departments and faculty should be identified, as this demonstrates commitment by the college. The people engaged and methods used in this follow-up should be identified. In some programs social media is used to engage students and to maintain contact with graduates. If this is the case with your program, you might indicate which social media will be used and who will be responsible for maintaining contact. Various programs use e-mail, social media, Facebook groups, online communities, and other easily accessible modes to maintain continuing contact with students. In addition, developing in students the habit of checking in and communicating with an online community and engaging program alumni with new students can build associations that will sustain connections. The National Student Clearinghouse can sometimes be helpful in maintaining information on program students.

CHAPTER SUMMARY

The Plan of Operation provides, in as much detail as page limits will allow, a road map to the implementation of the project. In most cases subsections specify the information required for the reader to ascertain the score to assign. The outline for the Plan of Operation section, including point values, is provided as an introduction to the chapter. Although the particular format for the Plan of Operation is from the TRIO selection criteria, this information has to be included in most proposals. In some RFPs the term "Plan of Operation" is not used as the title of the section, but in one form or another, the information outlined here must be provided. **I like to think of this section as a cookbook for conducting the project.** Each of the subsections—Plan to Inform; Plan to Recruit and Select Participants; Plan to Assess Individual Needs; Plan to Provide Services to Meet Identified Needs; and Plan to Manage the Project—is explained, and sample tables and charts are provided. This section of your proposal, in this case worth 30/100 points, is usually the longest and most detailed. The reader must see the connections among this section, the project's need, goals, and objectives, and the budget. Parts of the Master Table will be appropriately used in this section.

CHAPTER 13

Evaluation

- What is the purpose of the evaluation?
- What do the readers look for in my Evaluation section?
- Are there resources that will assist me in crafting a good evaluation?
- What is the difference between formative and summative evaluation?
- Which sections of the Master Table are in the Evaluation section?
- Do I need an external evaluator?
- Do I need to provide a research/evaluation design?
- What is a good research/evaluation design?
- What are the elements/factors/variables I need to consider in my design?
- What are the factors that might affect my research design?

The purpose of evaluation is to determine if your project is successful at achieving your goals/objectives for the population you are serving. The following is from the Federal Register Talent Search RFP

> Evaluation plan (8 points). The Secretary evaluates the quality of the evaluation plan for the project on the basis of the extent to which the applicant's methods of evaluation—
>
> **(1)** Are appropriate to the project's objectives;
>
> **(2)** Provide for the applicant to determine, using specific and quantifiable measures, the success of the project in—
>
> **(i)** Making progress toward achieving its objectives (a formative evaluation); and

(ii) Achieving its objectives at the end of the project period (a summative evaluation); and

(iii) Achieving its objectives at the end of the project period (a summative evaluation); and

(3) Provide for the disclosure of unanticipated project outcomes, using quantifiable measures if appropriate.

The evaluation section of your proposal provides an indication of how the project will be assessed to determine its success/achievement of the objectives. This section should be tied directly to the stated objectives and may include who will conduct the evaluation of the project, evaluation methods, data to be collected, research protocols, if any, to be used, and how the evaluation will be used to modify and improve the project. Both formative and summative evaluation processes should be used for all funded projects. A good introduction and overview of evaluation can be found at: **http://ww2.wkkf.org/digital/evaluationguide/main.html.** Practice exercises are included after Chapter 18.

Evaluation Overview

Evaluation is the systematic collection of data (qualitative and quantitative) throughout your project in order to determine that:

- The project is being conducted as described in the proposal (formative/process);
- Changes/modifications to the implementation of project activities and processes can be made in a timely fashion if needed; and
- The impact of project activities on participants can be assessed.

As noted in previous chapters, the evaluation shows how the activities you propose based on the needs of your participants result in changes in the measures you monitor to demonstrate short-term program outcomes. Table 13.1 is an excerpt from the Master Table. In the narrative to accompany this table, you will need to indicate:

- How many credits are needed for promotion to 10th grade;
- How you will define school attendance and how and how often you will get the numbers;
- How you will define and keep track of program attendance;
- How the GPA will be calculated;
- What are earned credits and how will you obtain them;

TABLE 13.1. Evaluation Process and Measures for Goals and Objectives

Need	Objective	Evaluative measures
Project Goal 1a: Increase the number/percent of low-income first-generation students completing 9th grade and entering 10th grade		
Low academic readiness for high school	95% percent of 9th grade program students will be promoted to 10th grade each year	School/program attendance, GPA, earned credits, individual course grades, credits earned in Summer Bridge to High School, Saturday Academy Program, and Before/After-School Tutoring, regents scores
Project Goal 1b: Increase the number of credits earned by low-income first-generation students entering 10th grade		
More than 50% of 9th-grade students are held over because they do not earn sufficient credits for advancement to 10th grade.	90% of program students will have 10 or more credits by the end of 9th grade.	School and program attendance, GPA, earned credits
Project Goal 1c: Increase the grade-point average earned by low-income first-generation 9th-grade students		
50% of student grades in the 9th grade are 65% or lower, revealing a lack of subject matter mastery needed for continued success.	85% of program students will show an increase in GPA of 5 percentage points by upper freshman term.	Program attendance, course grades, marking period, and semester GPA, teacher assessment of student learning

- How often you will monitor individual course grades (semester, marking period); the criteria for earning credits in program activities SBHS, SAPR, and B/AST) and how they will be counted by the school; and

- Which standardized test scores you will monitor.

A blank template is provided in Form 12.

Formative versus Summative Measures

Assessing the progress of your project and modifying activities and strategies as needed to assure that objectives are achieved is central to formative evaluation. The formative component includes qualitative and quantitative analysis of data gathered during the first 18–24 months of project implementation and is used to improve the project as it its implemented in its 3rd through 5th years. The majority of the objectives for the formative component are process oriented rather than outcomes oriented. The formative component should continue on a smaller scale during the 3rd through 5th years of project implementation to document fidelity to the final design of the project.

A specific section of the evaluation should address the formative evaluation and should include research/evaluation questions to be answered through the formative evaluation and a table that details the questions, data to be collected, and the timeline for collection.

Example of the Formative Evaluation Section

The *formative component* of the evaluation is used to establish baselines and to identify, modify, and/or create assessments to be used to track implementation and to measure the project's impact. An example is shown in Table 13.2. The research questions that will drive the formative evaluation are:

1. With what frequency does each of the proposed services (academic, professional development, induction, etc.) occur?

2. With what frequency and quality does collaboration between participants, staff members, faculty, and advisory boards occur?

3. How do the components of the organizational system supporting these proposed services integrate and function as a cohesive unit?

4. What kinds of experiences do the program participants and program staffs have as part of receiving/administering this program?

5. What is the perceived level of satisfaction of those receiving the proposed services?

6. What are service recipient's recommendations for service improvement?

7. What is the context in which this program is operating?

8. How and to what extent do contextual factors affect the provision of the proposed services?

9. What are specific, data-supported recommendations that can be made to program administration and staff in order to support the provision of high-quality services as defined by the project guidelines?

Example of the Summative Evaluation Section

This section is in response to the following, which expands and broadens, for clarity, one of the selection criteria discussed earlier: "(ii) Achieving its objectives at the end of the project period (a summative evaluation)."

The *summative component* of the evaluation should include, if feasible based on the number of participants and the availability of a comparison/control group, quasi-experimental and other quantitative statistical analyses to

TABLE 13.2. Formative Evaluation Activities, Data, and Timeline

Program activity	Type of data and method of collection	Timeline
1. *Reform* and implement an elementary education teacher preparation program	Review program materials Interview appropriate stakeholders (e.g., college faculty, school district and school administrators)	Beginning of project through end of first school year, continuing annually
2. Build school capacity to provide high-quality *clinical experiences* for preservice teachers	Interview college faculty and host school administrators Observe instances of the following: • Math and literacy discovery centers • PD for inservice teachers (year 1) • In-school activities of preservice teachers (years 2 and 3) • Interviews with preservice and inservice teachers	Spring or summer and continuing annually
3. Provide a sustainable, research-based, integrated *induction* program	Observe meetings of partnerships; participate in discussions of induction program activities. Observe development of video cases; view sample of videos produced	Years 1–5
4. Provide multilayered, coherent, relevant, and responsive *training and support* to all stakeholders	Review college teacher preparation program documents Observe "5th-year" activities of preservice teachers Interview college faculty, school personnel, and preservice teachers Observe instances of summer PD, PLCs, and induction activities	Onset of project through year 5
5. Engage in extensive *recruitment and rigorous selection* processes	Review recruitment documents Observe recruitment activities Interview participants Examine demographic data of participants	Years 1 through 3
6. Reform *literacy training* of preservice and inservice teachers to support the program focus	Observe instances of reformed training Review training documents and PD and induction program materials	Onset of project through year 3

Note. PD = professional development; PLC = professional learning communities.

determine whether project goals have been met. Most of the objectives of the summative component will be outcomes oriented.

The summative evaluation includes activities matched to the project goals and objectives. So in our example from the program presented in Chapter 11 and reproduced in Table 13.3, the objectives (expected outcomes) are presented along with the evaluative measures that will be used. In order to create this Table 13.3, all columns except those pertaining to objectives and evaluation have been removed, leaving a table in which the excerpted items match all other tables in which they appear.

In similar fashion to that shown in formative evaluation, you might pose a series of research/evaluation questions that highlight the summative evaluation elements.

1. What is the program impact on participating students' likelihood of graduation?

2. What is the program impact on participating students' short-term and long-term retention?

3. What is the impact of the program on student content knowledge in science?

4. What is the program impact on student entry into master's programs?

5. What is the immediate and long-term impact of the program on student achievement?

6. How do the attained outcomes compare when disaggregated (when possible) by grade level, race/ethnicity, gender, school, socioeconomic status, English language proficiency, or disability status of participants?

Another aspect of the evaluation narrative includes descriptions of surveys you will use, including reliability and validity, development and testing of surveys, questionnaires, observation forms, descriptions of data collection procedures, including who will collect data and how it will be stored, accessing college student data (enrollment, GPA, courses taken, credits earned); maintaining data files, confidentiality of the data that is collected and intention to file an institutional review board (IRB) application.

Evaluation Design

The evaluation design section details how the data you collect will be used to determine whether your project achieved the outcomes you proposed. If your knowledge of research/evaluation design is limited, you should consider working with someone within your institution with the skills to assist you. Alternately, if funds permit, you should consider hiring an evaluation consultant who

TABLE 13.3. Summary of Summative Objectives and Evaluative Measures from HSI-STEM Funded Proposal

Summative objectives	Evaluative measures
a. By September 2021 the number of enrolled Hispanic and low-income full-time STEM-field-degree-seeking undergraduate students will increase by 10% as compared to a control group.	• Number and percent of participant and nonparticipant undergraduate students in STEM. • Social belonging survey • Attendance at workshops • Enrollment in summer/winter classes
b. By September 2021 the number of retained first-time full-time STEM-field-degree-seeking undergraduate students who were in their first year of postsecondary enrollment in the previous year will increase by 10% as compared to a control group.	• GPA • Advisement sessions • Number of students identified through an Early Warning System • Attendance at workshops • Enrollment in summer/winter classes • Improvement in student perception in STEM
c. By September 2021 the number of Hispanic and low-income first-time, full-time degree-seeking undergraduate students enrolled at 4-year HSIs and graduating within 6 years of enrollment with a STEM field degree will increase by 10%.	• Credits earned • Time to graduation • Percent/no. of advisement sessions • Percent/no. of students identified with an Early Warning System • Attendance at workshops • Summer/winter enrollment • Use of academic support • Improvement in student perception of STEM
d. By September 2021 the number of Hispanic and low-income first-time, full-time degree-seeking undergraduate students enrolled at 2-year HSIs graduating within 3 years of enrollment with a STEM field degree/credential will increase by 10%.	• Attendance at workshops • Summer/winter enrollment • No. of advisement Sessions • Participation in REU • No./percentage of students on track to complete a degree • No./percentage of transfers to 4-year college
e. By September 2021 the number of Hispanic and low-income students transferring successfully to a 4-year institution from a 2-year institution and retained in a STEM field major will increase by 10% as compared to a control group.	• Number and percent of transfers to 4-year college • GPA overall and in STEM-related courses • GPA in gateway courses • Date of transfer evaluation and enrollment at 4-year college • Use of academic support
f., g., h., j. By September 2021 the number of Hispanic and low-income students participating in grant-funded student support programs or services, completing gateway courses in good academic standing, and completing a degree will increase by 10% as compared to a control group.	Number/percent of students: f. Participating in grant programs g. With Gateway course completion h. In good academic standing j. Completing a degree
i. By September 2021 the number of Hispanic and low-income STEM-field-major transfer students on track to complete a STEM field degree within 3 years from their transfer date will increase by 10% as compared to a control group.	• Credits earned • GPA • Time to degree • No./percent of students on track to complete a degree

is familiar with the program requirements of the funding agency. According to Graig (2012), an evaluation consultant should have technical competence, strong project management skills, excellent thinking skills, excellent ability to communicate with stakeholders, flexibility, and an orientation toward collaboration. In order to assess these competencies you need to consider the educational background of the evaluator (or the evaluation group), their evaluation experience as described on their website or in their literature, the length of time they have been in business, preliminary insights they have into your project and how to evaluate the outcomes, the services they will provide to the project as described by them, ease of communication, and responsiveness to inquiries. As many RFPs now require a response to invitational and/or competitive priorities, you may want to assess the consultant's willingness to help you develop responses and to suggest how the research identified can be used to inform the project design.

Research/Evaluation Design Basics

A research/evaluation design is a plan for collecting data and using it to assess your project. There are four designs used in evaluation: (1) pre-experimental designs, (2) experimental designs, (3) quasi-experimental designs, and (4) ex post facto designs. Before considering actual designs, it is useful to define the terms we will use (Rothstein, 1985).

- *Independent variable.* An independent variable is the treatment or intervention that is manipulated or varied. In your project some students may receive intrusive advisement while others may not. In this instance the independent variable is type of advisement and has two levels: intrusive advisement or standard advisement. The independent variable can also be called the treatment, and we might refer to the individuals who receive the treatment as the experimental group or treated group. Those who do not receive the treatment but instead have the status quo (standard advisement) are the control or untreated group.

- *Dependent variable.* This can be referred to as the measure referenced in your SMART objective; it is the variable that will change as a result of your independent variable. For example, students who receive intrusive advisement are expected to earn more credits or higher grades than students who receive standard advisement.

- *Subject variable.* In many cases it is useful to see whether your project activities have a differential impact on dissimilar types of individuals. Interesting comparisons can be drawn between males and females, urban and rural students, students of different ethnicities, ESL students versus native English speakers, and so forth. It will be especially useful to use a subject variable if you anticipate that the treatment may have differential impacts.

- *Comparison group.* Sometimes it is not possible to have an experimental group and a control group, so you may use a group of individuals who have attributes and characteristics similar to your participants but who are not part of the project to determine if your activities have an impact.

- *Extraneous intervening variables.* These are variables you may not be interested in or take into account in designing your project that can impact the relationship between the independent variables (project activities) and the dependent variables (measures) and influence the outcome of the project. We will see later that one way to control for extraneous variables is to use random assignment within an experimental design.

The research/evaluation design lays out the approach that will be used to determine how the activities/strategies/interventions you implement impact on achievement of the objectives you have proposed using the measures you have identified. In designing your approach prior research and theory play an important role. They inform the question development, design, analysis, and discussion phases of the project evaluation.

The Institute of Education Sciences (**https://ies.ed.gov**) and the WWC (**https://ies.ed.gov/ncee/wwc**) provide excellent resources for developing evaluations with examples of well-designed studies and reviews and summaries of studies that have met their stringent requirements.

In 1963 Campbell and Stanley published a book on research design in which they identified threats to both internal validity and external validity of research findings and suggested experimental designs that would alleviate these threats. Table 13.4 identifies the common threats to internal validity, and Table 13.5 identifies the common threats to external validity.

TABLE 13.4. Campbell and Stanley's (1963) Threats to Internal Validity

Threat	Description
History	Events other than the experimental treatments influence results.
Maturation	During the study, psychological changes occur within subjects.
Testing	Exposure to a pretest or intervening assessment influences performance on a posttest.
Instrumentation	Testing instruments or conditions are inconsistent, or pretest and posttest are not equivalent, creating an illusory change in performance.
Statistical regression	Scores of subjects that are very high or very low tend to regress toward the mean during retesting.
Selection	There are systematic differences between treatment groups in terms of subjects' characteristics.
Experimental mortality	Subject attrition may bias the results.
Diffusion of treatments	Implementation of one condition influences subjects in another condition.

TABLE 13.5. Campbell and Stanley's (1963) Threats to External Validity

Threat	Description
Reactive or interaction effect of testing	A pretest might affect performance on the posttest.
Interaction effects of selection biases and the experimental variable	Different participants might react differently to participation.
Reactive effects of experimental arrangements	Was the effect attributable to participation in the study?
Multiple treatment interference	Do multiple interventions produce unique effects?

There are two main approaches to a research problem—quantitative and qualitative methods. Quantitative methods are used to examine the relationship between variables with the primary goal being to analyze and represent that relationship mathematically through statistical analysis. This is the type of research approach most commonly used for scientific research problems. Qualitative methods are chosen when the goal of the research problem is to examine, understand, and describe a phenomenon. These methods are a common choice in social science research problems and are often used to study ideas, beliefs, human behaviors, and other research questions that do not involve studying the relationship between variables. Once the main approach to the research problem has been determined, several research designs may be considered for each type of approach.

These designs, whether used with qualitative or quantitative measures, can ameliorate the impact of these threats to internal and external validity. However it is not always possible to incorporate these "best" designs in a demonstration or programmatic project. These designs are summarized in Table 13.6.

TABLE 13.6. Common Research Designs

Design	Example	Drawbacks
Pre–post	G_1 O^1 X O^2	Does not account for extraneous or unidentifiable factors that might influence outcome
Two group	G_1 X O^2 G_2 O^2	No control for prior condition of group members
Two group pre–post	G_1 O^1 X O^2 G_2 O^1 O^2	No control for extraneous factors because no random assignment
Four group	G_1 O^1 X O^2 G_2 O^1 O^2 G_3 X O^2 G_4 O^2	Controls for the possible effect of the pretest but still no random assignment

Note. X, treatment; O^1, pretest; O^2, posttest; G, group.

Applying to the IRB for Human Subjects Research

Formal *review* procedures for *institutional* human subject studies were originally developed in direct response to research abuses in the 20th century, and any college or university that receives federal funding must have a formal IRB process. Individuals proposing to conduct research with human subjects must file an application prior to beginning their study. In order to facilitate this process, individuals are empaneled to review research protocols and related materials (e.g., informed consent documents and investigator brochures) to ensure protection of the rights and welfare of human subjects of research. Each investigator and any research assistants must complete an online certification to assure that they are fully versed in policies, rules, and regulations governing research with human subjects.

CHAPTER SUMMARY

The evaluation section presents an overview of a systematic process that indicates how you will know that the project is proceeding as described (formative or process evaluation) and how you will determine that you have achieved the proposed objectives (summative or product evaluation). The goals, objectives, and evaluation measures presented in the Master Table should match those presented here. For that reason I recommend that any changes to tables be made in the Master Table and then the tables for each section of the proposal be reformulated from the Master Table and reinserted into the appropriate section. In the narrative for the evaluation you would want to define any measures that are unusual and cite references for any published measures (surveys, demographic profiles, tests) you will use. It is also suggested that you have a separate section to describe the formative evaluation measures and clearly indicate that these are used to monitor the progress of the project and to make changes if warranted. A separate heading should be used for summative evaluation measures and should also indicate that yearly data will be reviewed to determine if goals and objectives are being met and if changes are warranted to assure they are met. If there are research questions or hypotheses that will be explored, then a section on the types of data (qualitative or quantitative) to be collected and the statistical (parametric or nonparametric) procedures used to analyze the data are presented in a separate section. Finally, if an outside evaluator will be contracted, you need to identify the person or evaluation firm and their credentials. The outside evaluator should have a significant role in shaping/writing the evaluation section of the proposal.

CHAPTER 14

Budget and Budget Narrative

LEARNING OBJECTIVES

- What are the elements of a budget?

- Who is the best person in my organization to help me with the budget?

- What is the best program to use in formulating a budget?

- What is a budget narrative?

- How many budget years do I have to provide?

- What are indirect costs?

- What are the federal or other budget forms I have to complete?

- How do I complete the federal or other budget forms?

The Budget Process

The project budget is an integral part of your proposal but must be able to stand on its own; that is, when reviewers look at the budget/budget narrative they should see a clear picture of the structure of the project. If you have never created a project budget or are unsure of what is included, I strongly recommend that you visit the Office of Research and Sponsored Programs (ORSP) as early as possible in the proposal-writing process. It is likely that they have sample budgets created for a wide range of funders and can assist you once you have an idea of the scope of the project. Practice exercises are included after Chapter 18.

There are two primary sections of any proposal budget: (1) *Personnel,* including who will be paid, rate of pay, time commitment, and total compensation (including fringe benefits based on the institution); and (2) *Other Than Personnel Services* (OTPS), which details all other costs for the project including travel, conference fees, materials, books, tests, consultants, and office supplies.

Other aspects of the budget include *indirect costs* mandated by your institution (a federally negotiated rate) or a funder-mandated rate and *participant*

163

stipends (usually exempt from indirect). The federally negotiated rate specifies what is included in the calculation of the amount permitted for indirect. There may also be other costs associated with your particular institution (New York City has the Metropolitan Transit Authority [MTA] tax on personnel costs).

Almost all funders also require the applicant to submit a budget narrative explaining who will be paid, the duties of each person/position, how and when they will carry out their duties, and the time commitment on an annual basis or for an academic year or summer.

So, a typical budget will have three sections (1) Personnel Costs, (2) OTPS Expenses, and (3) Indirect Costs. It is critical to check with your grants and contracts office early in the grant development process about submission and to ascertain whether anyone else in your organization is planning to apply for the same competition.

Personnel Costs

Fringe Benefits

Fringe benefits are forms of compensation provided to employees outside of wage or salary. Fringe benefits include medical and dental insurance, use of a company car, housing allowance, educational assistance, vacation pay, sick pay, meals, and employee discounts.

Each organization has salary schedules for personnel developed to recognize level of responsibility, current salary levels, and specific duties to be assigned. There are also specific fringe-rate percentages for full-time and part-time grant personnel. The rates are based on specific number of hours per week and benefits to be paid. The office that oversees grants and contracts in your institution or organization should be consulted to determine what the rules and regulations are governing salary levels, fringe rates, and other costs that must be included.

OTPS Expenses

Each RFP specifies the budget costs that are allowable and unallowable. Table 14.1 shows the allowable and unallowable costs for the TRIO program Talent Search. Other RFPs have additional unallowable costs. It is also useful, if you are not sure about whether a cost will be covered by the grantee, to contact your program liaison for clarification before the expense is incurred. The categories of transportation, testing materials, inservice training, space rental, computer and other equipment, and tuition costs are included.

Indirect Costs

Indirect costs are also termed administrative costs of the organization or institution hosting the program. These costs can be set for each institution through an analysis of documentation submitted on a regular basis by the institution. As noted previously, the proposal writer should check early and often with the

TABLE 14.1. Allowable and Unallowable Costs for Talent Search

Allowable costs*	Unallowable costs

(a) Transportation, meals, and, if necessary, lodging for participants and project staff for
  • Visits to IHEs
  • Participation in "College Day" activities
  • Field trips for participants to observe/meet with persons employed in various career fields who are role models for participants
  • Transportation to institutions of higher education, secondary schools not attended by the participants, or locations at which the participant receives instruction that is part of a rigorous secondary school program of study
	(a) Stipends and other forms of direct financial support for participants.

(b) Purchase of testing materials/test preparation programs	(b) Application fees for financial aid.

(c) Fees: admission applications for postsecondary education, college entrance examinations, or alternative education examinations if
  • A waiver of the fee is unavailable
  • Fee paid by grantee to third party on behalf of a participant
	(c) Research not directly related to the evaluation or improvement of the project.

(d) In-service training of project staff	(d) Construction, renovation, and remodeling of any facilities.

(e) Rental of space if
  • Space is not available at the site of the grantee
  • The space is not owned by the grantee	

(f) Purchase, lease, or rental of computer hardware, software, and other equipment, service agreements for such equipment, and supplies that support the delivery of services to participants, including technology used by participants in a rigorous secondary school program of study	
(g) Purchase, lease, service agreement, or rental of computer equipment/software for project administration/recordkeeping	

(h) Tuition costs for a course that is part of a rigorous secondary school program of study if
  • Course or a similar course is not offered at the secondary school attended by participant or another school within the school district
  • Grantee demonstrates that using grant funds is the most cost-effective way to deliver the course/courses necessary for completion of a rigorous secondary school program of study
  • Course is taken through an accredited institution of higher education
  • Course is comparable in content/rigor to courses that are part of a rigorous secondary school program of study as defined in § 643.7(b)
  • Secondary school accepts the course as meeting one or more of course requirements to obtain a regular secondary school diploma
  • Waiver of tuition costs is unavailable
  • The tuition is paid with Talent Search grant funds to an IHE on behalf of participant
  • The Talent Search project pays for no more than the equivalent of two courses for a participant each school year	

*Allowable costs must be reasonably related to the objectives of the project.

grants and contracts office; this is one category of information that is best provided by them. Sometimes the ORSP provides relevant proposal information on its website under the heading "Proposal Information" or has a summary available in the office. In your application you must report the negotiated indirect rate, the effective dates, and the government office issuing the rate. Many state and federal grantors and some foundation and corporate funders specify an indirect rate cap. For TRIO grants the indirect rate cap is 8%. Therefore, an institution can charge no more than 8% as an indirect cost.

Stipends and Other Expenses Not Subject to Indirect Costs

There are some costs that are not subject to indirect cost rate caps. These include student stipends, capital expenditures (if permitted by the RFP), and others. Again, your grants and contracts office will know which charges are subject to indirect cost caps and which are not. Figures 14.1, 14.2, and 14.3 present a series of screenshots from an actual budget. Please note that the column headings are D, F, H, J, L, and N. This is because the columns are used to calculate the fringe benefits are hidden. These columns are totaled and summarized in the shown columns in row number 83 for each column shown.

Microsoft Excel - budget submitted for HSI STEM and used in book without names

	A	B	C	D	F	H	J	L	N
1		HSI:STEM Budget		Year 1	Year 2	Year 3	Year 4	Year 5	Total
2				USDE	USDE	USDE	USDE	USDE	
3		Personnel							
4		Principal Investigators							
5			Vice President, Senior College (SC)						
6			Academic Dean, Community College 1 (CC1)						
7		Project Director							
8	0.38		TBD 100% T&E	$75,250	$76,755	$77,523	$78,298	$79,864	$387,689
9		Director (Campuses)							
10	0.38		Year 1 begin Feb 100% T&E	$36,300					$36,300
11	0.38		Year 2 to 5		$54,450	$54,995	$55,544	$56,100	$221,089
12		Academic Advisors							
13	0.38		1 @ 46,000/year 100% T&E	$46,000	$46,920	$47,389	$47,863	$48,820	$236,993
14	0.38		1 *19 hours/week x $35 x 40 weeks	$26,600	$26,866				$53,466
15	0.38		1 @ 46,000/year 100% T&E			$46,000	$46,460	$46,925	$139,385
16		Academic Support Coordinator							
17	0.10		19 hours/week x $35 x 40 weeks	$26,600	$26,866	$27,135	$27,406	$27,680	$135,687
18	0.10		19 hours/week x $35 x 40 weeks CC1	$26,600	$26,866	$27,135	$27,406	$27,680	$135,687
19	0.10		19 hours/week x $35 x 40 weeks CC2			$26,600	$26,866	$27,135	$80,601
20		Academic Coaches							
21			9 hours/week x $15 x 30 weeks						
22	0.10		Yr 1 2 at SC	$8,100					$8,100
23	0.10		Yr 1 1 at CC1	$4,050					$4,050
24	0.10		Yr 2 3 at SC		$12,150				$12,150
25	0.10		Year 2 2 at CC1		$8,100				$8,100
26	0.10		Yr 3 5 at SC			$20,250			$20,250
27	0.10		Yr 3 2 at CC1			$8,100			$8,100
28	0.10		Yr 3 1 at CC2			$4,050			$4,050
29	0.10		Yr 4-5 6 at SC				$24,300	$24,300	$48,600
30	0.10		Yr 4-5 2 at CC1				$8,100	$8,100	$16,200
31	0.10		Yr 4-5 2 at CC2				$8,100	$8,100	$16,200
32		Career Advisor							

Sheet1 Sheet2 Sheet3

Type here to search

FIGURE 14.1. Screenshot of the first 32 lines of the submitted budget for a grant showing a section of the personnel costs as well as the fringe rates used by applicant.

Microsoft Excel - budget submitted for HSI STEM and used in book without names

	A	B	C	D	F	H	J	L	N
33	0.10		19 hours/week X $35 X 40 weeks x $35 SC		$26,600	$26,866	$27,135	$27,406	$108,007
34		**Admin Assoc/Data Entry and Analysis**							
35	0.38		Yr 1 50% T&E	$30,000					
36	0.38		Yr 2-5		$60,600	$61,206	$61,818	$62,436	$246,060
37		**Research Liaison**							
38	0.51		Academic Year 11% T&E ($150,812)	$16,390	$16,554	$16,554	$16,554	$16,554	$82,607
39	0.26		Summer 1 month	$15,176	$15,328	$15,328	$15,481	$15,636	$76,949
40		**Faculty Team Leaders**							
41	0.26	Summer Salary SC 15 x $3000		$18,000	$18,000	$18,000	$18,000	$18,000	$90,000
42	0.26	Summer Salary CC14 X $4,500		$18,000	$18,000	$18,000	$18,000	$18,000	$90,000
43	0.26	Summer Salary CC2 4 X$4,500				$18,000	$18,000	$18,000	$54,000
44		**Staff Team Leaders**							
45	0.095		4 x5 hours/week x 20 weeks x $45	$18,000	$18,000	$18,000	$18,000	$18,000	$90,000
46	0.095		4 x5 hours/week x 20 weeks x $45	$18,000	$18,000	$18,000	$18,000	$18,000	$90,000
47	0.095		4 x5 hours/week x 20 weeks x $45			$18,000	$18,000	$18,000	$54,000
48		**Faculty Professional Development**							
49	0.095		Workshop Leader 50 hours X $200	$10,000	$10,000	$10,000			$30,000
50	0.26	Faculty Summer Salary 15 x $3000		$45,000					$45,000
51	0.26	Faculty Summer Salary 15 x $3000			$45,000				$45,000
52	0.26	Faculty Summer Salary 15 x $3000				$36,000			$36,000
53	0.1	Instructors Winter Sessions 6 x $4,500		$27,000	$27,000	$27,000	$27,000	$27,000	$135,000
54	0.1	Instructors Summer Sessions 6 x $4,500		$27,000	$27,000	$27,000	$27,000	$27,000	$135,000
55	0.095	Tutors Yr 1 14 X 14 X 100 hours SC		$19,600					$19,600
56	0.095	Tutors Yr 1 6 X 14 X 100 hours CC1		$8,400					
57	0.095	Tutors Yr 2 17 X 14 X 100 hours SC			$23,800				$23,800
58	0.095	Tutors Yr 2 6 X 14 X 100 hours CC1			$8,400				$8,400
59	0.095	Tutors Yr 3 17 X 14 X 100 hours SC				$23,800			$23,800
60	0.095	Tutors Yr 3 6 X 14 X 100 hours CC1				$8,400			$8,400
61	0.095	Tutors Yr 3 6 X 14 X 100 hours CC2				$8,400			$8,400
62	0.095	Tutors Yr 4 & 5 17 X 14 X 100 hours SC					$23,800	$23,800	$47,600
63	0.095	Tutors Yr 4 & 5 6 X 14 X 100 hours CC1					$8,400	$8,400	$16,800
64	0.095	Tutors Yr 4 & 5 6 X 14 X 100 hours CC2					$8,400	$8,400	$16,800

Sheet1 / Sheet2 / Sheet3

FIGURE 14.2. Screenshot of lines 33 to 64 of the submitted budget showing personnel costs section which follows that shown in Figure 14.1.

Microsoft Excel - budget submitted for HSI STEM and used in book without names

	A	B	C	D	F	H	J	L	N
65	0.095		Peer Mentor Training 30 X 20 hrs X $18	$10,800	$10,800	$10,800	$10,800		$43,200
66	0.095		Peer Mentoring 30 X50 hours X $18		$27,000	$27,000	$27,000	$27,000	$108,000
67		**Total Salaries and Wages**		$530,866	$622,055	$718,530	$684,731	$679,336	$3,235,518
68		**MTA**		$1,545	$1,854	$2,212	$2,219	$2,200	$10,030
69		**Total Fringe Benefits**		$122,887	$145,446	$168,569	$159,877	$158,998	$755,778
70		**Total Personnel**		$655,298	$769,354	$889,311	$846,828	$840,534	$4,001,325
71		**Other than personnel services**							
72		**Travel**							
73			PD to Required Meeting	$3,000	$3,000	$3,000	$3,000	$3,000	$15,000
74			Professional Staff to Required Meetings	$7,000	$7,000	$7,000	$7,000	$7,000	$35,000
75		**Supplies & Materials**							
76			Lab/Research/Admin/Student Materials fo	$80,000	$53,452	$30,000	$40,000	$20,000	$223,452
77			Lab/Research/Admin/Student Materials fo	$50,000	$40,000	$15,000	$20,000	$10,000	$135,000
78			Lab/Research/Admin/Student Materials for CC2		$40,000	$15,000	$20,000	$10,000	$85,000
79		**Computers for Staff 10 X $1,200**		$12,000					
80		**Software 10 X $402.70**		$4,027					
81		**Ipad Minis for Students**		$37,275	$40,979	$23,283	$22,719	$19,553	$143,807
82		**Contractual Evaluators**		$75,000	$50,000	$50,000	$50,000	$75,000	$300,000
83		**Total OTPS**		$268,302	$234,431	$143,283	$162,719	$144,553	$953,286
84		**Total Direct**		$923,600	$1,003,785	$1,032,593	$1,009,546	$985,087	$4,954,611
85		**Indirect yr 8%**		$73,888	$80,303	$82,607	$80,764	$78,807	$396,369
86		**Student Stipends**		$50,000	$80,000	$80,000	$105,000	$120,000	$435,000
87		**Total Project Costs**		$1,047,488	$1,164,088	$1,195,201	$1,195,310	$1,183,894	$5,785,980
88		**Allocated by HIS:STEM**		$1,047,488	$1,164,088	$1,195,201	$1,195,310	$1,183,894	$5,785,981
89									
90									
91									
92									
93									
94									
95									
96									

Sheet1 / Sheet2 / Sheet3

FIGURE 14.3. Screenshot of lines 65 to 88 of the submitted budget showing remaining personnel costs, summary of personnel costs, fringes and personnel totals, followed by the other than personnel services (OTPS), the total direct costs, indirect costs, student stipends, total project costs, and the amount allocated by the funder.

Sample Budget Narrative

Your proposal is required to have a detailed budget narrative for each year of the project. Every expense must be described and justified. The budget narrative presented in Table 14.2 is for year 1 of a proposed HIS:STEM proposal. In some cases, if costs are higher than might be anticipated, they should be justified by average costs in your organization and reasons why it may be necessary to have higher salaries to attract fully qualified applicants for project positions. Table 14.2 presents the budget narrative for the first year of the project. The RFP states that a narrative budget must be submitted for each year of the proposal. The format will be the same but some of the information might change by year.

CHAPTER SUMMARY

An initial budget should be drafted with a fiscal manager (grants and contracts office, treasurer, accountant, chief financial officer) early in the proposal development process because the budget you present with your proposal must coincide with the personnel, fringe benefits, materials, equipment, and supplies you propose to use for the activities provided to participants. Although the budget section is usually worth only a few points (5 or so), loss of even these points can make the difference between making the funding cut or missing it. The budget needs to be reviewed and likely revised several times during the proposal-writing process, so creating a spreadsheet using formulas is highly recommended. RFPs always have a section on what expenses are allowed and what expenses are disallowed. If you budget for expenses that are disallowed, the funder probably will not let you revise the budget to move the funds elsewhere—they will just award less. The budget narrative needs to provide detail on how each expense amount was determined. For personnel, include full-time/part-time, hours worked, weeks worked, rate of pay, fringe benefits, and a brief summary of responsibilities (excerpted from the table in the Plan of Operation). For OTPS, details needs to include what you are purchasing, how many, and the per-item cost. For books and materials, the per-item cost should be multiplied by number of participants The more detail provided in the budget narrative, the better judgment the reader/funder can make.

TABLE 14.2. Sample Budget Narrative

<u>BUDGET NARRATIVE FOR YEAR 1</u>

HSI-STEM: Pathways to STEM Success—Using High-Impact Practices to Improve STEM Enrollment, Retention, Transfer, and Graduation

<u>Year 1 Personnel</u>

Project Investigators (PIs)—7% Time and Effort, covered by the colleges	
Vice President for Enrollment Management, SC **Associate Dean of Academic Affairs, CC-1** **Dean of Academic Affairs, CC-2 (Year 3)**	

The Project Investigators (PI) in Years 1 and 2 are the Provost for Enrollment Management and the Associate Dean of Academic Affairs for Curriculum Matters and Faculty Development CC-2. In Year 3 the Dean of Academic Affairs from CC-3 will join the team. The PIs will be responsible for managing the project and meeting with the Steering Committee and the Advisory Board. They will host meetings with the evaluation team. Project administrators will join the team in Year 3.

Project Director (PD) —100% Time and Effort	**$75,250**

The Project Director (PD) will be responsible for the day-to-day operations of the project and will report to the PIs. The PD will be responsible for oversight and evaluation of project staff and will chair the Advisory and Steering Committees. The PD will meet regularly with the staff team leaders.

Director of Campuses (DC)—100% Time and Effort (8 Months) in Year 1	**$36,300**

The Director of Campuses (DC) will be the liaison between the SC and the CC-1 and CC-2 and will be responsible for the day-to-day operations at the community colleges. He or she will report to the PD and will meet regularly with the CC PIs. The DC will serve on the Advisory and Steering Committees and will work with the Faculty and Team Leaders at each community college campus.

Academic Advisors	
Advisor 1–100% Time and Effort	**$46,000**
Advisor 2—Part-Time	**$26,600**

The Academic Advisors will be responsible for implementing the intrusive advising model. The 100% advisor will begin at Lehman and will meet with the part-time advisor, who will begin at CC-1. In Year 3 when CC-2 is added the part-time advisor will become full-time.

Academic Support Coordinators (2)	
19 hours per week × $35 × 40 weeks SC	**$26,000**
19 hours per week @ $35 × 40 weeks CC-1	**$26,000**

Each campus in the project will have a part-time Academic Support Coordinator. The SC coordinator will have 19 hours per week beginning in Year 1; the CC-1 coordinator will have 19 hours per week beginning in Year 1.

Academic Coaches (3)	
9 hours per week × $15 × 30 weeks × 2 AC	**$8,100**
9 hours per week × $15 × 30 weeks CC-1	**$4,050**

In Year 1 the project will begin with four Academic Coaches, two at SC and two at CC-1. In Year 2 there will be eight coaches, four at SC and four at CC-1. Numbers will increase until Year 4, when there will be a total of 12 coaches across the three campuses.

(continued)

TABLE 14.2. *(continued)*

Career Advisor	

The Career Advisor (CA) for the project will not begin until Year 2. Using the substantial resources of the career advisement center the CA will meet regularly with groups and individual participants to share the resources available for career exploration and also offer frequent workshops on success in college, careers in STEM, internship opportunities, connecting with faculty members, and setting goals and objectives for college/careers.

Administrative Associate and Data Entry and Analysis	
Year 1—50% Time and Effort	$30,000

The administrator, data entry, and analysis individual will work closely with the Administrative Coordinators, the Project Director, the Research Liaison, and the Evaluators, assuring that fiscal reports, expenditures, and payments are tracked. The bulk of the time will be devoted to maintaining a project database with current student information. This person will also work with the college registrar to maintain and download participant files from the University and College databases.

Research Liaison	
Academic Year—11% Time and Effort ($150,812)	$16,390
Summer—1 Month	$15,176

The Research Liaison has experience working with external evaluators and maintaining and using databases with large college projects. He or she will work with the data analyst and with the evaluators to assure that data for the project are available as needed.

Faculty Team Leaders	
4 from SC × $4,500 and 4 from CC-1 × $4,500	$36,000

The faculty team leaders will be drawn from the STEM departments at the participating colleges. They will meet regularly to review/discuss the activities of the project and to recommend modifications, changes, and additions. In particular, they will review the development/progress of the Research Experiences for Undergraduates and the incorporation of active learning components in classrooms. They will also review the faculty development activities. Team Leaders will be added from CC-2 in Year 3.

Staff Team Leaders	
4 × 5 hours per week × 20 weeks × $45 SC	$18,000
4 × 5 hours per week × 20 weeks × $45 CC-1	$18,000

The Staff Team Leaders will be drawn from the administrative departments of admissions, advisement, curriculum, and academic support, and from the School of Natural and Social Sciences at the participating colleges. They will meet regularly to review/discuss the activities of the project and to recommend modifications, changes, and additions. In particular, they will review the development/progress of the admission and transfer processes and the coordination among the administrative offices at the SC and community colleges. Staff Team Leaders will be added from CC-2 in Year 3.

Faculty Professional Development	
Workshop Leader—50 hours × $200	$10,000
Faculty Participants Summer Salary—15 × $3,000	$45,000

A workshop leader will be responsible for developing and delivering project director for faculty participating in the project. Topics will be selected after a survey of faculty and staff team leaders and participating faculty.

(continued)

TABLE 14.2. *(continued)*

Instructors	
6 courses Winter Session	**$27,000**
6 courses Summer Session	**$27,000**

Participating students will be provided the opportunity to enroll in needed courses and intensive mathematics sessions and participate in REU opportunities during winter sessions and summer sessions. Students who require additional credits or need to make up a gateway course will also have the opportunity to enroll. This initiative is based on the finding that students who complete 15 credits per semester and 30 credits per year will have a greater chance of graduation.

Tutors for Academic Support	
14 × 14 × 100 hours SC	**$19,600**
6 × 14 × 100 hours CC-1	**$8,400**

Academic tutors and mentors will work under the auspices of the Academic Support Coordinator to provide assistance to participants during semester, winter and summer courses.

Personal Peer Mentors (Selection and Training)	
30 × 20 hours × $18	**$10,800**

Personal Peer Mentors have been used with great success in introductory and gateway chemistry courses. During Year 1 a total of 30 Peer Mentors will be selected and trained. The training takes 20 hours and engages Peer Mentors in workshops and supervised work with students. They will work one on one with students in gateway science courses to assure comprehension, understanding of concepts, success in assignments, and high grades.

Total Salaries and Wages	*$530,866*
Metropolitan Transit Authority Surcharge on Wages	*$1,545*
Fringe Benefits	*$122,887*
Total Personnel	*$655,298*
Other Than Personnel Services (OTPS)	
Travel	
PD to Required Meetings	**$7,000**
Professional Staff to Required Meetings	**$3,000**

Enable the PD to attend required and training project meetings accompanied by selected professional staff. Will cover travel, hotel, local travel, and per diem.

Lab/Research/Administrative/Student Supplies and Materials	
Supplies and Materials for SC	**$80,000**
Supplies and Materials for CC-1	**$50,000**

Participating colleges will require funds for laboratory materials for students, student supplies, books, award recognition, certificates, materials for students, and some administrative costs for faculty and staff teams and for Advisory Board meetings. Each college's allocation decreases over years.

(continued)

TABLE 14.2. *(continued)*

Computers with Software for Staff	
10 × $1,200	**$12,000**
10 × $402.70	**$4,027**

Up to 10 staff members will require a computer to perform the duties of their positions. Either desktop or laptop for use with students, in meetings with other staff and for report writing, accessing student data, and submitting data. The cost of software for each computer is $42.70.

iPads for Students	
75 × $497	**$37,275**

iPads will be available for students to use in classes, in conjunction with their Research Experience for Undergraduates and to access online textbooks and other electronic resources. All courses at Lehman include an online component so students must be able to access BlackBoard and to submit their work. Finally, students will be able to take notes more easily in class with an iPad.

Contractual Evaluators	**$75,000**

The project will employ an external evaluator who will be involved in the design of the evaluation, design and assist with the selection of evaluative measures, administer or assist in administering measures to assess student outcomes, gather data with the assistance of the Data Administrator and the Research Liaison. Our external evaluator will receive a total of $300,000 over the 5-year period of the grant. The full amount of the negotiated contract with the evaluator will be paid unevenly over the 5 years; the first payment is the largest.

Total OTPS	**$268, 302**
Total Direct	**$923,600**
Indirect (Restricted Rate = 8%)	**$73,888**
Student Stipends (Not Included in the Indirect Calculation)	**$50,000**

Student stipends will be calculated based on class level (freshman, sophomore, junior, or senior); type of research project; time devoted to research; and staff recommendations. The amount available will increase each year.

Total Project Costs	**$1,047,488**

Note. CC-1 = community college 1; CC-2 = community college 2; SC = senior college.

PART III

Additional Considerations

CHAPTER 15

Dissemination, Sustainability, and Significance

Dissemination

Dissemination means informing others about the results of the project or research. The degree of emphasis placed on dissemination in the proposal is dependent upon the guidelines of the funding agency and the type of project. A published report or article may be necessary. Perhaps regional or local workshops are to be given. A manual or guide for curriculum may be sent to teachers.

In writing about dissemination of your project findings, you want to provide information to the reader on the kinds of information you will freely share with or make available to others. This can include curricula, lesson plans, activity descriptions, PowerPoints, data and outcomes, or videos. You also want to indicate with whom you will communicate—individuals such as other researchers, other projects, community members, future students, participants, faculty, or the general population. What are the potential implications for those with whom you will share outcomes and activities? How will you share your information? This can include research publications, general publications in professional journals, presentations at conferences (locally, regionally, nationally, internationally), professional development days, or classes and speeches. How will you know if your dissemination efforts are well received?

Dissemination may be accomplished in one or more of the following ways: conferences, curriculum guides, seminars, newsletters, on-site visits for professionals, media releases, working papers, articles in journals, presentations, pamphlets, books or manuals, audiovisual materials. model courses or curricula, inservice training programs, self-instructional materials, and demonstrations of techniques.

Dissemination can be implemented through a website for your program that is linked to the website of the institution in which your project is located. Elements of the website should include several tabs that feature a description/abstract of your program; pictures of participants (if you have obtained photo releases) engaged in project activities; descriptions of some of the activities; resources that you have used or that can be used by others for similar programs; links, for program students and staff, to useful websites, forms, and releases for program application/participation; applications for program-sponsored events, information for parents/guardians, and pictures and descriptions of events; and, most important, accomplishments of participants in the program (graduation, entrance into postsecondary education, completion of dual enrollment courses, community service, human interest stories, and individual student work).

Sustainability

Think of project funding as providing the opportunity to implement practices that have the potential to make a difference for your institution and the individuals it serves and that could not be "tested" within the annual budget. The additional funding pays for trying out these promising strategies and practices to determine if they make a difference for your students, institution, faculty, or administration.

Most grants are funded over several years (5 years is usual). This gives the institution time to evaluate the processes and outcomes on a yearly basis (and to submit an annual report to the funder with outcomes and milestones) and to modify strategies, activities, and methods that are not working as well as anticipated. Funders realize that even the best ideas need time to be developed and tweaked to be successful and the funded institution is expected to do just that. So by the third year you have a model that produces the short-term results you proposed.

Often, institutions propose to increase future outcomes, including graduation rates, application and entry to higher levels of education, and entry into careers. These cannot be measured in 1 year so, as we saw in the evaluation section, the proposal should include participants entering at different levels so that goals are achieved during the project. A well-designed and through evaluation will determine which activities, strategies, and services have the greatest impact on achievement of project goals and objectives.

Funders want to know that the work they have supported will be sustained after their funding ends. They anticipate that best practices will be institutionalized and continue to positively impact the institution and its students. This can be accomplished by transitioning project personnel to institutional positions over the life of the project; adopting strategies, materials, and methods that have proven successful in meeting project goals; and integrating program elements into ongoing work.

Strategy to Scale

Strategy to scale is a different way of asking about project sustainability. The RFP for HSI-STEM includes specific questions about scaling the project. The guidelines from Title 34—Education 75.210 general selection criteria are shown here:

(1) The Secretary considers the applicant's strategy to scale the proposed project.

(2) In determining the applicant's capacity to scale the proposed project, the Secretary considers one or more of the following factors:

(i) The applicant's capacity (e.g., in terms of qualified personnel, financial resources, or management capacity) to bring the proposed project to scale on a national or regional level (as defined in 34 CFR 77.1(c)) working directly, or through partners, during the grant period.

(ii) The applicant's capacity (e.g., in terms of qualified personnel, financial resources, or management capacity) to further develop and bring to scale the proposed process, product, strategy, or practice, or to work with others to ensure that the proposed process, product, strategy, or practice can be further developed and brought to scale, based on the findings of the proposed project.

(iii) The feasibility of successful replication of the proposed project, if favorable results are obtained, in a variety of settings and with a variety of populations.

(iv) The mechanisms the applicant will use to broadly disseminate information on its project so as to support further development or replication.

(v) The extent to which the applicant demonstrates there is unmet demand for the process, product, strategy, or practice that will enable the applicant to reach the level of scale that is proposed in the application.

(vi) The extent to which the applicant identifies a specific strategy or strategies that address a particular barrier or barriers that prevented the applicant, in the past, from reaching the level of scale that is proposed in the application.

Significance

Funders are making an investment in change for the better. You need to convince them (and the reader) that the strategies and activities they are supporting will make a difference at your institutions, in the community, and for your partners. Each of the selection criteria listed here focuses on an aspect of this expectation (Federal Register, 2009):

> The Secretary considers the significance of the proposed project. In determining the significance of the proposed project, the Secretary considers the following factors:
>
> **(i)** The likelihood that the proposed project will result in system change or improvement.
>
> **(ii)** The extent to which the proposed project is likely to build local capacity to provide, improve, or expand services that address the needs of the target population.
>
> **(iii)** The importance or magnitude of the results or outcomes likely to be attained by the proposed project, especially improvements in teaching and student achievement.
>
> **(iv)** The potential for continued support of the project after Federal funding ends, including, as appropriate, the demonstrated commitment of appropriate entities to such support.

The example provided is a shortened version of a section from a proposal prepared for the Teacher Quality Partnership Program (Lehman College, 2010).

(i) The likelihood that the proposed project will result in system change or improvement.

The lessons learned through this project will be used to improve/reform all programs within the Division of Education. This will be the first fifth-year program at the college and the first to engage preservice teachers in a stipended ½-day, 5-day-per-week on-site fieldwork. Data show that its diverse pool of undergraduates minoring in teacher education fail to persist to certification because of financial and family constraints that prohibit taking a semester off from undergraduate study to student teach.

The proposed fifth-year program better meets the needs of student from underrepresented groups to obtain both initial and professional certification with a combined BA/MA program that respects their need for employment to support their families. Thus, the program is the first to respond to the needs of the diverse, borough resident student population of the college. It will also be the first program working with the city education department to provide a 2-year induction program for graduates that collaborates with school personnel. Further, the program provides a model of school-focused, needs-based preparation program development that develops knowledge and skills along a continuum from preparation through induction that is responsive, rigorous and consistent with district priorities and school needs. The digital content developer, a local cable provider, will prepare video cases to document processes and materials that can be utilized to impact further teacher preparation program reform within the partnership, across the university and shared with other teacher education programs. While this is not the first program that uses the cohort model, this initiative extends the model to place a subcohort of preservice teachers at each of five host schools.

Thus, over the 5 years of this program, the program reforms will be documented, sustained, and integrated into additional programs leading to institutionwide reform. Program reforms to be replicated include rigorous admissions of students from underrepresented groups, cohort supportive structures and monitored progress through the program of study, development of capacity at host school sites, co-teaching with school personnel, extended clinical experiences (½ day, 5 days per week from September to June), school-based courses, and needs-based curriculum design in collaboration with the local education authority (LEA) in which program emphases are integrated with LEA priorities, the assessment process for preservice teachers is aligned with its identified qualities, and preparation to use data through its database is provided to teachers.

The initiative has the potential to provide systemic improvement in the collaborative nature of the program model between schools and teacher preparation programs and among higher education faculty, school personnel, and recognized experts in evaluation, professional development, and mathematics. Historically at odds, the school-focused, needs-based design of the initiative brings together schools and higher education with a common goal that is made real through a focus on student achievement through the continuum of teacher development preparation programs, professional development, and induction.

(ii) **The extent to which the proposed project is likely to build local capacity to provide, improve, or expand services that address the needs of the target population.**

There are three areas of potential impact on local capacity: the capacity of the schools to serve as demonstration sites for best practices, the capacity of an institution of higher education to respond to local needs in program development, and the capacity of both entities to collaboratively improve the preparation, competence, and retention of teachers.

To build local capacity in the schools, the initiative proposes to develop Math Discovery Centers within each host school so that the schools have centers in which to study (through inquiry groups and professional learning communities) the development of mathematical learning in elementary-age urban children. These centers then also serve as demonstration sites for best practices in instruction and assessment. Furthermore, the initiative engages cooperating teachers in professional development in the content focus of the proposed program as well as training student teacher mentors prior to the placement of participants in the schools. This yearlong preparation of host school sites builds their capacity as collaborative partners in teacher preparation.

The college will, through the program, build its capacity to prepare and provide teachers for local schools who are representative of the ethnic and linguistic populations of their neighborhoods. Further, capacity for developing school-focused, needs-based teacher preparation programs is enhanced with school personnel involvement in program course delivery, integration of adjunct and full-time faculty into professional development and induction support, involvement of school personnel in program management, and alignment of the content of the teacher preparation program with LEA priorities and initiatives. Lastly, the collaboration of the schools and the institution of higher education will build capacity for long-lasting improvement in recruitment, retention, and competency practices.

Teachers are recruited who are from the neighborhoods in which they will teach and, as research shows, are more likely to stay in teaching as a result. Furthermore, teacher competency and a focus on student achievement are congruent between the graduate program of study and the clinical experience, professional development, and induction segments of the program. This focus on shared ownership of teacher preparation builds local capacity to continue to engage at this high level of simultaneous reform. The initiative's project design underscores the value of a shared ownership process to sustain responsibility for the collaborative model after the funding period ends.

(iii) The importance or magnitude of the results or outcomes likely to be attained by the proposed project, especially improvements in teaching and student achievement.

The innovative design for is a fifth-year program focused on preparing early childhood and childhood teachers with an emphasis on content and pedagogy in mathematics constitutes a system change and synergizes the capacities of complimentary educational institutions. The program includes (1) having participants spending ½ days in a host school, selected with the collaboration of LEA, observing and working with a cooperating teacher; (2) preparing teachers to teach mathematics, within the context of early child and childhood settings, to a diverse urban, largely bilingual and special needs population; (3) offering courses co-taught by education faculty/math specialists and teachers from host schools; (4) implementing an extensive, focused 2-year induction program with mentoring, professional development, and summer seminars involving school colleagues; and (5) developing a series of early childhood and childhood visual mathematics case studies for student analyses and professional development.

The importance of program reform in teacher preparation and its potential replication in the borough and beyond, however, are not enough. Preparing borough residents as teachers for local schools means that borough students and families will finally be able to see themselves in the classrooms in which they learn. *That* has the potential to transform student motivation and attendance as well as teacher turnover. Developing best practices at sites in one of the poorest areas in the United States means that where urban diversity and challenges are urgently real, so is the potential for excellence in teaching and learning. *That* has the potential to transform urban neighborhoods and a cycle of undereducation and poverty. Bringing together the talents and expertise of personnel in public schools, public higher education, and private entities means that this is not "their" problem, it is *our* challenge. *That* has the potential to transform business as usual. If we can make a difference here, in our borough, we can make it anywhere. And the more models we, as a nation, have for reducing the achievement gap and for improving teacher preparation, the more likely we are to eliminate the "shame" of a society that can build a space shuttle and, yet, fail to educate all of its citizenry to the same level of excellence.

(iv) The potential for continued support of the project after Federal funding ends, including, as appropriate, the demonstrated commitment of appropriate entities to such support.

Continued support for the reforms developed and piloted through the initiative will be pursued during the grant period. The reformed program of study will be registered with the state education department and will become the first early childhood/childhood mathematics fifth-year certification program in the university. Additional programs will be reformed as evidence of program impact becomes available through formative evaluation and research studies and the video cases created by the local cable provider will ensure that preparation training processes and tools are sustained. Demonstration site development will be documented and replication will be instituted at the discretion of the LEA. To sustain the program stipends provided during clinical experience, supplemental financial support will be pursued through the LEA as the program shows impact and effectiveness. The LEA currently allocates millions of dollars to the preparation of alternative route teachers with its teaching fellows programs as well as support for the Teach for America program. When the proposed program demonstrates positive outcomes, LEA financial support for teacher preparation in shortage areas will find support. As additional students are admitted, program tuition revenues, enrollment numbers, and university and grant supplemental funding will sustain further reforms and innovations of the teacher preparation programs at the college. Program participants will seek TEACH grant and federal funding for graduate study.

CHAPTER SUMMARY

Funders want assurance that your project outcomes will inform the practice and/or research of other similar institutions/organizations. A section that indicates the ways in which the outcomes of your project will be disseminated/

shared with others should include possible and planned publications, presentations, website postings, expansion to others, and use of training opportunities. It is also critical to indicate that the activities of the project will not end when funding ends, but that they will be institutionalized or sustained within your organization. Often, external funding is used to test the efficacy of changes in how outcomes are achieved. Once new approaches are found to be successful, it is assumed that they will be implemented in place of the previous approaches. Finally, you need to provide evidence of the significance of your project. Significance can encompass both sustainability and dissemination, but on its own it refers to the extent to which your project can enhance the capacity to address the community or organizational needs identified in Section 1 of your proposal.

CHAPTER 16

Addressing Invitational and Competitive Priorities

Over the past decade the USDE has required that proposals address invitational and competitive priorities and provide research evidence to support the activity to be implemented. **Absolute priorities** describe items that a proposal must address in its application in order to receive an award. Reviewers determine if the priorities are met after evaluating the proposer's response to all of the Selection Criteria. Funding will be awarded only for applications that meet the absolute priorities. **Invitational priorities** signal areas the USDE is particularly interested in; applicants may choose to address one or more of the invitational priorities. Applicants who meet an invitational priority do not earn extra points and are not given preference over other applications. A **competitive preference priority** describes an area of particular interest for which an applicant may earn additional points. Proposers should respond to the competitive preference priority throughout their application. However, each competitive priority must be addressed with supporting evidence from studies approved by the Institute for Education Sciences. Specific references must be cited and connections between the research presented and the proposal's strategies and activities must be provided. Absolute priority does not carry any value but must be addressed in order to be chosen for funding. The invitational priority does not carry any point value but as it represents areas of high interest to the USDE the proposer should make an effort to address it in the proposal. However, the competitive priority does carry a point value. Responding to the competitive priority is optional, but proposers who fail to respond are at a distinct disadvantage. RFPs that offer competitive priorities specify the number of additional pages a proposal is allowed to address each competitive priority included. These are in addition to the page limitations provided and are included with the proposal. A list of the 15 areas identified in the *Federal Register* is presented in Table 16.1.

In 2014 the USDE released, through the *Federal Register* (Vol. 79, No. 237, December 10, 2014, pp. 73426–73456), a compendium of the potential competitive priorities that might be used in RFPs. As the proposer's response to each competitive priority must be supported by research that meets the evidence conventions of the IES's What Works Clearinghouse (WWC), it can be useful to read the detailed definition for each area of interest, which is presented in the full compendium. Table 16.1 provides only the title for each area, but the specific page number in the *Federal Register* is also provided if you want to access the full definition. Practice exercises are included after Chapter 18.

TABLE 16.1. *Federal Register* **Listing of Competitive Priorities for USDE Grants**

Priority	Title	Page
I	Improving Early Learning and Development Outcomes	73429
II	Influencing the Development of Non-Cognitive Factors	73430
III	Promoting Personalized Learning	73431
IV	Supporting High-Need Students	73433
V	Increasing Postsecondary Access, Affordability, and Completion	73433
VI	Improving Job-Driven Training and Employment Outcomes	73435
VII	Promoting Science, Technology, Engineering, and Mathematics (STEM) Education	73436
VIII	Implementing Internationally Benchmarked College- and Career-Ready Standards and Assessments	73438
IX	Improving Teacher Effectiveness and Promoting Equitable Access to Effective Teachers	73439
X	Improving the Effectiveness of Principals	73441
XI	Leveraging Technology To Support Instructional Practice and Professional Development	73442
XII	Promoting Diversity	73444
XIII	Improving School Climate, Behavioral Supports, and Correctional Education	73445
XIV	Improving Parent, Family, and Community Engagement	73446
XV	Supporting Military Families and Veterans	73447

As a rule, both invitational and competitive priorities must use research that produces at least moderate evidence of effectiveness as defined by the IES guidelines and analysis. This chapter takes you through a process that will enable you to completely and accurately answer the invitational and competitive priorities. The moderate evidence of effectiveness required to support the activities to be implemented in your project can be obtained by a search of the WWC website. Frequently, the RFP will suggest research studies approved by the WWC that meet the criteria for evidence of effectiveness.

Both invitational and competitive priorities are included in RFPs published in the *Federal Register,* and their inclusion must be noted in your application. An example of how this requirement appears in the RFP is provided below.

> Priorities: This notice contains one competitive preference priority and one invitational priority. In accordance with 34 CFR 75.105(b)(2)(ii), the competitive preference priority is from 34 CFR 75.226. Applicants must include in the one-page abstract submitted with the application a statement indicating if they addressed the competitive preference priority and/or the invitational priority.
>
> Competitive Preference Priority: For FY 2017 and any subsequent year in which we make awards from the list of unfunded applications from this competition, this priority is a competitive preference priority. Under 34 CFR 75.105(c)(2)(i), we award three additional points to an application that meets this priority.
>
> Applications that address one or both of the priorities are instructed as follows:
>
> . . . any application addressing the competitive preference priority may include up to four additional pages, and any application addressing the invitational priority may include up to two additional pages. The additional pages allotted to address priorities cannot be used for or transferred to the application narrative or any other section of the application. Applicants addressing the competitive preference priority and/or the invitational priority should include them in a separate section of the application submission and discuss how the application meets the competitive preference priority and/or the invitational priority.

Rules Governing Evidence for Invitational and Competitive Priorities

A presentation of the types of evidence required for supporting the activities you must or will choose to implement under these priorities can be found in the Educational Regulations section 75.226 This section (34 CFR 77.1(c)) provides the definitions and types of research needed.

> What procedures does the Secretary use if he or she decides to give special consideration to applications supported by strong evidence of effectiveness, moderate evidence of effectiveness, or evidence of promise?
>
> **(a)** As used in this section, "strong evidence of effectiveness" is defined in 34 CFR 77.1(c);

(b) As used in this section, "moderate evidence of effectiveness" is defined in 34 CFR 77.1(c);

(c) As used in this section, "evidence of promise" is defined in 34 CFR 77.1(c); and

(d) If the Secretary determines that special consideration of applications supported by strong evidence of effectiveness, moderate evidence of effectiveness, or evidence of promise is appropriate, the Secretary may establish a separate competition under the procedures in 34 CFR 75.105(c)(3), or provide competitive preference under the procedures in 34 CFR 75.105(c)(2), for applications supported by:

(1) Evidence of effectiveness that meets the conditions set out in either paragraph (a) or (b) of the definition of "strong evidence of effectiveness" in 34 CFR 77.1(c).

Strong evidence of effectiveness means one of the following conditions is met:

There is at least one study of the effectiveness of the process, product, strategy, or practice being proposed that meets the What Works Clearinghouse Evidence Standards without reservations, found a statistically significant favorable impact on a relevant outcome (with no statistically significant and overriding unfavorable impacts on that outcome for relevant populations in the study or in other studies of the intervention reviewed by and reported on by the What Works Clearinghouse), includes a sample that overlaps with the populations and settings proposed to receive the process, product, strategy, or practice, and includes a large sample and a multi-site sample.

> **(a)** There are at least two studies of the effectiveness of the process, product, strategy, or practice being proposed, each of which: Meets the What Works Clearinghouse Evidence Standards with reservations, found a statistically significant favorable impact on a relevant outcome (with no statistically significant and overriding unfavorable impacts on that outcome for relevant populations in the studies or in other studies of the intervention reviewed by and reported on by the What Works Clearinghouse), includes a sample that overlaps with the populations and settings proposed to receive the process, product, strategy, or practice, and includes a large sample and a multi-site sample.

(2) Evidence of effectiveness that meets the conditions set out in the definition of "moderate evidence of effectiveness;" defined in 34 CFR 77.1(c); Moderate evidence of effectiveness means one of the following conditions is met:

> **(a)** There is at least one study of the effectiveness of the process, product, strategy, or practice being proposed that meets the What Works Clearinghouse Evidence Standards without reservations, found a statistically significant favorable impact on a relevant outcome (with no statistically significant and overriding unfavorable impacts on that outcome for relevant populations in the study or in other studies of the intervention reviewed by and reported on by the What Works Clearinghouse), and includes a sample that overlaps with the populations or settings proposed to receive the process, product, strategy, or practice.

(b) There is at least one study of the effectiveness of the process, product, strategy, or practice being proposed that meets the What Works Clearinghouse Evidence Standards with reservations, found a statistically significant favorable impact on a relevant outcome (with no statistically significant and overriding unfavorable impacts on that outcome for relevant populations in the study or in other studies of the intervention reviewed by and reported on by the What Works Clearinghouse), includes a sample that overlaps with the populations or settings proposed to receive the process, product, strategy, or practice, and includes a large sample and a multi-site sample.

(3) Evidence of effectiveness that meets the conditions set out in the definition of "evidence of promise" defined in 34 CFR 77.1(c)

"Evidence of promise" means there is empirical evidence to support the theoretical linkage(s) between at least one critical component and at least one *relevant outcome* presented in the *logic model* for the proposed process, product, strategy, or practice. Specifically, evidence of promise means the conditions in both paragraphs (i) and (ii) of this definition are met:

(a) There is at least one study that is a—

(i) Correlational study with statistical controls for selection bias;

(ii) Quasi-experimental design study that meets the What Works Clearinghouse Evidence Standards with reservations; or

(iii) Randomized controlled trial that meets the What Works Clearinghouse Evidence Standards with or without reservations.

(b) The study referenced in paragraph (i) of this definition found a statistically significant or substantively important (defined as a difference of 0.25 standard deviations or larger) favorable association between at least one critical component and one relevant outcome presented in the logic model for the proposed process, product, strategy, or practice.

For a recent Upward Bound competition the invitational priority was:

Moderate Evidence of Effectiveness (3 points).

Applications supported by evidence of effectiveness that meets the conditions set out in the definition of "moderate evidence of effectiveness" in 34 CFR 77.1(c).

Invitational Priority: For FY 2017 and any subsequent year in which we make awards from the list of unfunded applications for this competition, this priority is an invitational priority. Under 34 CFR 75.105(c)(1), we do not give an application that meets this invitational priority a competitive or absolute preference over other applications. The Secretary encourages applicants to propose projects designed to increase opportunities for participants to earn postsecondary credits in high school, such as through providing connections to dual enrollment programs.

For a recent Upward Bound Math and Science competition the competitive priority was:

> This notice includes a competitive preference priority that encourages applicants to propose activities that are supported by moderate evidence of effectiveness (as defined in this notice). The Department is particularly interested in receiving applications that include plans to provide services for students, supported by evidence, that increase the likelihood that students will complete high school and enroll in and complete a program of postsecondary education. The Department is not specifying a particular service, such as tutoring or mentoring, that is tied to evidence, but is providing an opportunity for the applicant to decide which statutorily authorized service the project will implement based on available evidence of effectiveness.
>
> Definitions: These definitions are from 34 CFR 77.1.
>
> Moderate evidence of effectiveness means one of the following conditions is met:
>
> **(i)** There is at least one study of the effectiveness of the process, product, strategy, or practice being proposed that meets the What Works Clearinghouse (WWC) Evidence Standards without reservations, found a statistically significant favorable impact on a relevant outcome (with no statistically significant and overriding unfavorable impacts on that outcome for relevant populations in the study or in other studies of the intervention reviewed by and reported on by the WWC), and includes a sample that overlaps with the populations or settings proposed to receive the process, product, strategy, or practice.
>
> **(ii)** There is at least one study of the effectiveness of the process, product, strategy, or practice being proposed that meets the WWC Evidence Standards with reservations, found a statistically significant favorable impact on a relevant outcome (with no statistically significant and overriding unfavorable impacts on that outcome for relevant populations in the study or in other studies of the intervention reviewed by and reported on by the WWC), includes a sample that overlaps with the populations or settings proposed to receive the process, product, strategy, or practice, and includes a large sample and a multisite sample.
>
> Relevant outcome means the student outcome(s) (or the ultimate outcome if not related to students) the proposed process, product, strategy, or practice is designed to improve; consistent with the specific goals of a program.

"What Works Clearinghouse Evidence Standards" means the standards set forth in the WWC *Procedures and Standards Handbook* (Version 3.0, March 2014).

Research areas covered by the WWC standards are literacy, mathematics, science behavior, children with disabilities, English learners, teacher excellence, dropout prevention, early childhood, kindergarten through 12th grade, path to graduation, and postsecondary. Clicking on each of these areas will provide studies that have been reviewed and will indicate whether they meet any one of the three levels of evidence as defined in 34 CFR 77.1.

Responding to Invitational and Competitive Priorities

When the USDE first began to implement the invitational and competitive priorities and to require evidence of effectiveness, there were suggested studies included that met the criteria for moderate evidence of effectiveness. I believe that this was to help organizations understand what was intended. In recent RFPs this has not been the case. So let's go through a process you might use to identify qualifying research studies for a few invitational and competitive priorities.

Finding Evidence for a Dual Enrollment Program

Dual enrollment programs exist under many different names in almost all states, and recent studies producing moderate evidence of effectiveness, as well as some monographs, are available through the WWC. The WWC uses the IES review processes to establish evidence of effectiveness. If you access the WWC home page and click on Path to Graduation (see Figure 16.1a), you will see Dual Enrollment Programs among the list in the screen that comes up next (Figure 16.1b). The orange graduation hat to the left shows that there are research studies providing evidence supporting the dual enrollment intervention. When you click on Dual Enrollment Programs, you can see details about the actual studies that were reviewed for level of evidence (Figure 16.1c), including the number of studies that met WWC standards for various areas of focus (called "outcome domains") and other information.

If we click on the first outcome domain, Access and Enrollment, we find four studies that each have some evidence of effectiveness: Berger, Garet, Hoshen, Knudson, and Turk-Bicakci (2014); Edmunds et al. (2015); Giani, Alexander, and Reyes (2014); and Struhl and Vargas (2012).

In formulating the response to the invitational priority, we would provide a brief overview of the four studies and would then describe how the program we are proposing (the same dual enrollment program described in the next section) would use the methods of dual enrollment described in these articles and why we would expect our program outcomes to be similarly effective.

In looking at each study, we note the following: Berger et al. (2014) were studying an early college high school initiative. We realize that our program is not located in a similar setting. Some of the characteristics of the program are similar to ours: college-credit courses were taught by college instructors; minority student enrollment was over 50%, first-generation and low-income student enrollment was high, and half of the schools were in urban settings. Although reported results support dual enrollment, perhaps one or more of the other studies will be more similar to our project.

The second study, by Edmunds et al. (2015), also considers the impact of the early college model. They followed several cohorts of North Carolina Early

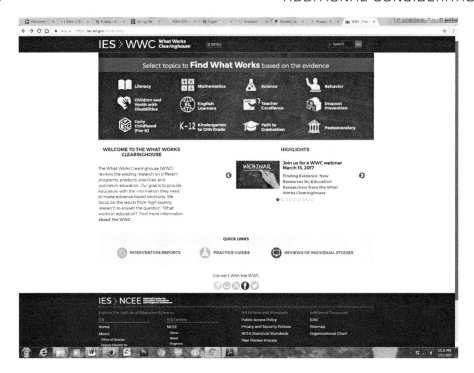

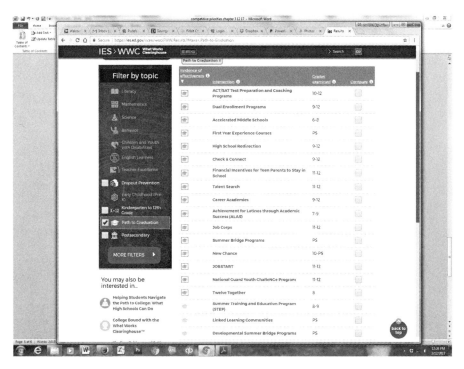

FIGURE 16.1. Screenshots of the home page for the What Works Clearinghouse and citations for college readiness.

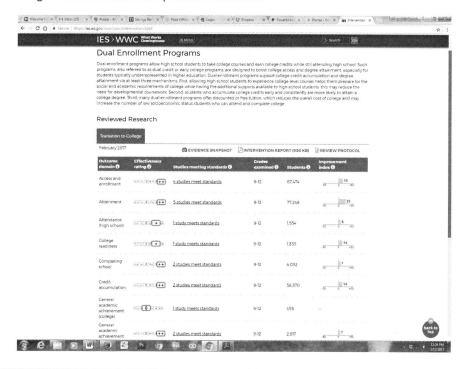

FIGURE 16.1. *(continued)*

College students through high school and high school graduation into college and college graduation. As in the previous study, comparisons with a random control group showed that the early college program had a supportive positive impact on students.

The third study, by Giani et al. (2014), explored variations in the impact of dual-credit coursework on postsecondary outcomes. The dual-credit coursework significantly impacted college access, persistence, and college completion. However, means were not provided.

Struhl and Vargas (2012) followed the impact of dual enrollment on high school students in Texas in conjunction with Jobs for the Future. They suggest that allowing students to experience real college coursework through dual enrollment is one of the best ways to prepare them for college. In this study they followed high school graduates for 6 years beyond graduation and found that students who experienced a college course were 50% more likely to earn an associate or higher degree from a Texas college within 6 years compared to students who did not participate. In order to account for the fact that students who take dual enrollment courses may be stronger students, the comparison group was comprised of students matched using a propensity score match.

So, by using studies that were reviewed by the IES and presented in the WWC, we can show that the activity/practice we plan to implement has had a significant impact on student enrollment in and graduation from college.

Example of an Invitational Priority Response

Invitational Priority: Dual Enrollment Program

The dual enrollment program to be employed in the Upward Bound Program is the successful CUNY-wide College Now Program, which offers free tuition and books to junior and senior high school students who qualify (75% on the English and math regents). College Now students can enroll for up to 16 college credits prior to high school graduation.

Dual enrollment programs allow students to take college courses and earn college credits while still attending high school. These programs have been shown to boost college access and degree attainment, especially for students typically underrepresented in higher education (What Works Clearinghouse Intervention Report, 2017). Dual enrollment programs support college credit accumulation and degree attainment via at least three mechanisms: high school students experience college-level courses and prepare for the social/academic requirements of college with additional supports available to them; students accumulate college credits early and are more likely to attain a college degree; and many dual enrollment programs offer discounted/free tuition, reducing the cost of college and increasing the number of students at a low socioeconomic level who can attend and complete college.

The *What Works Clearinghouse Intervention Report* (2017) included five studies with at least moderate evidence that reported that dual enrollment programs had positive effects on students' degree attainment (college), college access and enrollment, credit accumulation, high school completion, and general academic achievement (high school), with a medium to large extent of evidence. Of the five studies that met WWC design standards, only the three who met the standards with reservations studied dual enrollment. All of them used quasi-experimental designs.

The most relevant to our program was An (2013), which studied the effectiveness of a dual enrollment program using data from the National Education Longitudinal Study. The intervention group was comprised of 2,000 students who attended postsecondary school and participated in a dual enrollment program. The comparison group attended postsecondary school but did not participate in a dual enrollment program. Several variables known to be related to college outcomes were selected for matching.

An (2013), Giani et al. (2014), and Struhl and Vargas (2012) demonstrated that dual enrollment programs were effective and that participating students were more likely to stay in high school, be ready for college, and have good high school attendance. An's (2013) study also explored the effect of taking one, two, or more than two courses. He found that students who enroll in two or more courses are more likely to attain a BA than nonparticipants. Most students who enroll in College Now at Lehman take 6–12 credits. The three studies that considered the impact of dual enrollment used criteria for selecting the intervention group that is consistent with our programs. The studies reviewed did not note whether there were specific qualifications for enrolling in their programs. The criteria that the College Now program uses are consistent with entrance requirements to CUNY colleges. Lehman College has been tracking the outcomes for dual enrollment students for about 15 years and in that time has noted that dual enrollment students tend to persist, take more credits each semester, and earn higher grade-point averages than students who do not take dual enrollment courses. So our results are similar to those of the studies reviewed (An, 2013; Giani, Alexander, & Reyes, 2014; Struhl & Vargas, 2012; WWC Intervention Report, 2017).

Example of a Competitive Priority Response

Competitive Priority: Mentoring Program

Carrell and Sacerdote (2013) examined the impact of college application coaching on high school seniors. The program they report on was aimed at senior students whose school counselors believed they were unlikely to apply to college despite sufficiently high scores to qualify. They used random assignment. The intervention group received the college coaching program, which was implemented by college students and provided in-person assistance with completing college application and financial aid forms, money to cover application fees, and a $100 cash incentive to participants for completing the college application process. The primary outcome of interest was whether students enrolled in college and attended at least three semesters of college. Women assigned to the treatment group see large (15 percentage point) increases in their college-going rate and these differences persist through at least the second year of college. The treatment appears to move some women from attending 2-year colleges to 4-year colleges and some from no college to a 2-year or a 4-year college. The researchers found that the intervention had no significant impact on men.

The assessment of why men did not react as women did raises some interesting questions. Carrell and Sacerdote (2013) suggest that men respond differentially (or even negatively) to advice or indirect feedback while women might infer that they are better prepared or suited for college than they previously believed. Men may infer that they are in the program because they are less prepared or less capable then they thought. Finally, the authors opine that the treatment could be correcting or compensating for some lack of personal confidence or lack of family attention experienced by the women but not the men.

This proposal suggests a strong mentoring program with all of the elements mentioned by Carrell and Sacerdote with the exception of the cash incentive. In addition, we begin working with students in their sophomore year to assess college readiness, share information on financial planning and budgeting for college (with groups of students and their parents), introduce them to the FAFSA application and assist them in completing it, begin to assist them with choosing an appropriate college, hold college fairs, schedule college visits, and make college information available. One of the incentives we offer is that students who do well can qualify to take college credit courses through Lehman and earn as many as 12 college credits, saving them one semester of college tuition and book and material costs and fees.

Although Sinclair, Christenson, Evelo, and Hurley (1998) and Sinclair, Christenson, and Thurlow (2005) studied youth with disabilities, their work focused on reducing dropping out of school. It is based on monitoring of school performance, mentoring, case management, and other supports. The "Check" component is designed to continually monitor student performance and progress. The "Connect" component involves program staff giving individualized attention to students in partnership with other school staff, family members, and community service organizations.

Our program includes elements of check and connect, as students are assigned a school counselor advocate who meets with them regularly in individual and group sessions, reviews attendance, class cutting, behavior, and academic progress and checks in with their teachers regularly; when needed the school counselor advocate intervenes by contacting teachers or parents. He or she also advocates for assigned students, coordinates services, provides ongoing feedback and encouragement, emphasizes the importance of staying in school, and assists students in college awareness and preparation.

The role of the school counselor advocate as a mentor is enhanced by our program's use of Facebook and other social media. Students, counselors, and the project director can communicate regularly through the project accounts. It also enables former program participants now in college to communicate with the program staff on a regular basis and to reach out to current participants, as our program graduates came from the same schools we are now serving and may know the current juniors and seniors.

For example, in one of our after-school programs we found it difficult to get students to come after school for tutoring services, especially if they were satisfied with their grades (even though they were very low). Most students only came to tutoring if they were failing a class and required to attend. We needed to motivate the students to come to the after-school program and to work harder to increase their GPAs. In the second year, we hired upperclassmen to tutor and mentor the lowerclassmen. The peer tutors/mentors also assisted in the recruitment for the after-school program. Overall, students were more receptive to hearing the benefits of the program from other students, were able to see their peers in positions of leadership, and were motivated to excel by the chance to be hired for the program. This gave students the motivation to work harder and come to tutoring. Since implementing the peer mentoring program, we have been able to meet our enrollment objectives every year. Students who show success continue to be hired by the program. Students look up to their peers and envision themselves completing high school and entering college like their mentors. Peer mentoring increased the number of students applying to college; however, the number of students actually enrolling in college still remained low. To help increase the number of students enrolling in college, we took the mentoring program one step further and added college students to the program. The college students who joined the mentoring program were successful Lehman College undergraduates who are enrolled in the TRIO Student Support Services Program, Careers in Teaching. As a further step, we developed a mentoring program handbook (Palmieri, 2016) so that all mentors understand their role and duties. Mentor training activities include identifying a past mentor and thinking about how he or she helped; discussing the possible roles of a mentor; understanding what a good mentor does and does not do; guidelines; program procedures for mentors; mentoring stages; mentoring myths; presentation guidelines; and sample lessons and activities (Carrell & Sacerdote, 2013; Palmieri, 2016; Sinclair, Christenson, & Thurlow, 2005).

CHAPTER SUMMARY

For the past decade or more, funders have asked that proposals include responses to invitational and competitive priorities. Invitational priorities are not associated with scoring, but competitive priorities can earn from 1 to several extra points for the proposal. Both of these priorities require that applicants use evidence to support the activity/activities they will implement in addressing them. The cited research must meet WWC Evidence Standards (**https://ies.ed.gov/ncee/wwc**). Invitational priorities must be met in order for the proposal to be considered, but competitive priorities are optional. However, the opportunity to earn extra points should not be passed up, as it could make a difference in whether the funding cut score is achieved.

CHAPTER 17

Guide to Proposal Review and Scoring

Each funding agency, corporation, or foundation has a method of reviewing and scoring proposals as well as a way of determining which proposals will be funded. Federal agencies have the most transparent method, as the review and scoring criteria are often presented in the selection criteria section of the RFP. Table 17.1 presents review criteria from a USDE Student Support Services RFP and the point values the reviewer is to use for each one.

Each reviewer who is empaneled reads 8–10 proposals and scores them using the common scoring system. These readers generally log in to eGrants or Grants.gov to access their assigned proposals and then enter their scores and comments into the system once they have evaluated the proposal.

What Happens When You Submit Your Proposal?

As we have seen, you submit your proposal through Grants.gov, eGrants, or a portal used by your college, agency, or school district. Once you submit it, the proposal is date-verified and reviewed for errors (Does the information match what is on file? Does the agency name match the DUNS (Data Universal Numbering System) number? Does the format match the required guidelines?)

TABLE 17.1. Review Criteria and Point Values

			Point value
a.	Need for the project		24
	1.	Number or percentage of students who meet eligibility requirements	8
	2.	Academic and other problems eligible students encounter	8
	3.	Differences between eligible and noneligible SSS/PTS students	8
b.	Objectives		8
	1.	The extent to which project participants persisted toward completion of the academic programs in which they were enrolled	3
	2.	The extent to which project participants met academic performance levels required to stay in good academic standing at the grantee institution	2
	3.	The extent to which project participants graduated	3
c.	Plan of Operation		30
	1.	Informs the institutional community (students, faculty, and staff)	3
	2.	Identifies, selects, and retains project participants with academic need	3
	3.	Assesses each individual participant's need and monitors academic progress	4
	4.	Provides services that address the goals and objectives of the project	10
	5.	Ensures proper and efficient administration of the project	10
d.	Institutional commitment		16
	1.	Committed facilities, equipment, supplies, personnel, and other resources	6
	2.	Established administrative and academic policies	6
	3.	Demonstrated commitment to minimizing dependence on student loans	2
	4.	Assured full cooperation/support of admissions, student aid, registrar, and IR	2
e.	Quality of personnel		9
	1.	The qualifications required of the project director	3
	2.	The qualifications required of other project personnel	3
	3.	The quality of the applicant's plan for employing personnel who have succeeded in overcoming barriers similar to those confronting the project's target population	3
f.	Budget		5
g.	Evaluation plan		8
	1i.	Appropriate to the project—includes both quantitative and qualitative evaluation	2
	1ii.	Examines the success of the project in improving academic achievement, retention, and graduation of project participants	2
	2.	Uses evaluation results to make programmatic changes	4

Following recent problems concerning dismissing Upward Bound applications for minor formatting errors, it is not clear whether or how any future formatting regulations will be enforced. My take on this is that the need to adhere to a page limit forces the writer(s) to be more concise and targeted in the narrative and may result in a better proposal.

Who Reads Your Proposal?

Your proposal is read by a panel of at least three individuals assisted by a USDE staff member who convenes the group at regular intervals during the review process to discuss the proposals, their strengths and weaknesses, the scoring, and the total scores. The readers have all applied for their positions through the USDE using the following link to the Field Reviewer System: **www.g5.gov**. In order to use the G5 system you must sign up. Doing it now will facilitate using it in the future. Participating as a grant reviewer helps you learn about the grant process, become familiar with a grant program and/or funding agency, learn about innovations that are being proposed, and meet colleagues and funding agency representatives in your field. It is by far the best way to learn about developing grant proposals. Each reader is expected to thoroughly review each assigned proposal and provide comments in each scored section to point out strengths and weaknesses that led to the assigned score.

What Is the Scoring System and How Are Points Awarded?

The scoring system is based on assignment of a predetermined (and legislated) value to each element of the proposal. Table 17.1 shows the total values for each section as well as its component values. So, for example, the Plan of Operation, as shown, is worth 30 points. A complete answer on informing the institutional community is worth 3 points, as is the information on how you will identify, select, and retain participants who demonstrate academic need. Your description of how you will assess participant need and monitor progress is worth 4 points. Comprehensive and complete responses in these sections are likely to be less detailed than those in the final two components, each of which is worth 10 points.

For the fourth and fifth components of this section, you will want to use clear tables and charts (think Master Table, Chapter 6). In the case of component 4 ("provide services that address the goals and objectives of the project"), you can use a table to present the goals and objectives of the project along with the services/activities that will achieve them. Also critical in this section is to show how the schedule of activities will relate to the objectives and a description of the activities to be implemented.

For component 5 ("Ensure proper and efficient administration of the project"), you need to include tables that present timelines, organizational figures, and the qualifications, roles, responsibilities, and time commitments of key personnel.

How Is Funding Determined?

Once all of the submitted proposals are scored and the reviewer totals are summed and averaged, program liaisons (in the case of TRIO grants) add prior experience points for each submitting institution (explained below) to the average for each proposal, and the proposals are placed in order by score from the highest to the lowest. Funding begins with the top-ranked proposal and continues down the list until all available funds are allocated.

What Are Prior Experience Points?

Previously funded programs that are applying for a grant are eligible to receive prior experience points based on previous project performance and added to the total external reviewer score. In this way programs that continue to be successful are more likely to receive funding than programs applying for the first time.

Prior experience points are awarded on the basis of the specific objectives that needed to be met by each program and on whether the program met or exceeded the targeted percentage required for each of the objectives. In the recent Upward Bound Proposal guidelines that our college responded to, these objectives, as presented in this application, were:

> Objectives (9 points). The Secretary evaluates the quality of the applicant's objectives and proposed targets (percentages) in the following areas on the basis of the extent to which they are both ambitious, as related to the need data provided under paragraph (a) of this section, and attainable, given the project's plan of operation, budget, and other resources:
>
> 1 Academic Performance—Grade Point Average (GPA)
>
>   _____% of participants served during the project year will have a cumulative GPA of 2.5 or better on a 4-point scale at the end of the school year.
>
> 2 Academic Performance on Standardized Test Tests
>
>   _____% of Upward Bound seniors served during the project year will have achieved at the proficient level on state assessments in reading/language arts and math.
>
> 3 Secondary School Retention and Graduation
>
>   _____% of project participants served during the project year will continue in school for the next academic year, at the next grade level, or will have graduated from secondary school with a regular secondary school diploma.

4 Secondary School Graduation (rigorous secondary school program of study)

_____% of all current and prior year Upward Bound participants who graduated from high school during the school year with a regular secondary school diploma will complete a rigorous secondary school program of study.

5 Postsecondary Enrollment

_____% of all current and prior UB participants who graduated from high school during the school year with a regular secondary diploma will enroll in a program of postsecondary education by the fall term immediately following high school graduation, or will have received notification by the fall term immediately following high school from an institution of higher education of acceptance but deferred enrollment until the next academic semester (e.g., spring semester).

6 Postsecondary Completion

_____% of participants who enrolled in a program of postsecondary education by the fall term immediately following high school graduation, or by the next academic term (e.g., spring term) as a result of acceptance by deferred enrollment, will attain either an associate or bachelor's degree within 6 years following graduation from high school.

Your program liaison uses the middle 3 years of your project (2, 3, 4) to determine the extent to which you achieved aspects of your project as indicated in your proposal (Code of Federal Regulations, 2018).

The Department calculates prior experience points from data submitted in annual performance reports (APRs). Achievement rates for each PE criterion will be based on the project's approved objectives and on the information the grantee provided in the APR for each assessment year under consideration. (U.S. Department of Education, 2017)

For purposes of the PE [prior experience] evaluation of grants awarded after January 1, 2009, the Secretary evaluates the applicant's PE on the basis of the following outcome criteria:

(3 points) *Number of participants.* Whether the applicant provided services to no less than the approved number of participants.

(1.5 points) *Academic performance.* Whether the applicant met or exceeded its approved objective with regard to participants served during the project year who had a cumulative GPA at the end of the school year that was not less than the GPA specified in the approved objective.

(1.5 points) Whether the applicant met or exceeded its approved objective with regard to participants served during the project period who met the academic performance levels on standardized tests as specified in the approved objectives.

(3 points) *Secondary school retention and graduation.* Whether the applicant met or exceeded its approved objective with regard to participants served during

the project year who returned the next school year or graduated from secondary school with a regular secondary school diploma.

(1.5 points) *Rigorous secondary school program of study.* Whether the applicant met or exceeded its approved objective with regard to current and prior participants with an expected high school graduation date in the school year who completed a rigorous secondary school program of study.

(3 points) *Postsecondary enrollment.* Whether the applicant met or exceeded its approved objective with regard to current and prior participants with an expected high school graduation date in the school year who enrolled in a program of postsecondary education within the time period specified in the approved objective.

(1.5 points) *Postsecondary completion.* Whether the applicant met or exceeded its approved objective with regard to participants who enrolled in a program of postsecondary education and attained a postsecondary degree within the number of years specified in the approved objective (U.S. Department of Education, 2017)

Figure 17.1 (pp. 202–205) is a blank reader comment form for a recent Student Support Services competition. The reader has to identify the strengths and weaknesses of each section and then assign a point value. Figure 17.2 (pp. 206–216) is a completed reader review from the same competition that represents one reader's scoring of Lehman College's most recent Student Support Services proposal.

Note that all proposal scoring is completed online so that the reviewers can enter their review after each of the criteria.

CHAPTER SUMMARY

One of the best opportunities for honing your proposal-writing skills is to become a peer reviewer. The USDE encourages individuals to submit their profile and provides a site (**www2.ed.gov/about/offices/list/ope/trio/ seekingfieldreaders.html**) where you can apply to read, for example, TRIO proposals. You can also become familiar with the peer review process by studying the forms used to score proposals. You will see that they exactly follow the selection criteria for the proposal and include score values as well as fields for the reviewer to indicate the strengths and weaknesses of the proposal.

APPLICATION TECHNICAL REVIEW FORM
(READER'S COMMENT FORM)
STUDENT SUPPORT SERVICES
LAST UPDATED January 5, 2015
34CFR PART 646.21(SELECTION CRITERIA)

Applicant   Application Number

Descriptive Name of Project

Address

INSTRUCTIONS: This form is furnished for your use in evaluating the attached application. Please complete all pages and return the entire form to us; be as thorough and explicit as possible in your responses. We are requesting your professional evaluation of the applicant's need for the project, strengths and weaknesses of their plan to address these needs through the proposed project, and their plans to evaluate the project's success. If you have any questions concerning the application, please contact the program officer assigned to your panel.

SUMMARY RATINGS

	MAXIMUM POINTS	SCORE
1. NEED	24	_____
2. OBJECTIVES	8	_____
3. PLAN OF OPERATION	30	_____
4. INSTITUTIONAL COMMITMENT	16	_____
5. QUALITY OF PERSONNEL	9	_____
6. BUDGET	5	_____
7. EVALUATION PLAN	8	_____
TOTAL		_____

COMPETITIVE PREFERENCE PRIORITIES 1a (1 point), 1b (2 points)

2a (1 point), 2b (2 points)   (6 points)   _____

TOTAL Maximum Score for Selection Criteria and Competitive Priority   106 points   _____

APPLICATION TECHNICAL REVIEW FORM

NOTE: Readers MAY be instructed to list "Strengths and Weaknesses" for each criterion to which points are attached and for the total application.

(a) NEED FOR THE PROJECT: (24 points) [646.21(a)]
The Secretary evaluates the need for a Student Support Services project proposed at the applicant institution on the basis of the extent to which the application contains clear evidence of:

(1) (8 points) A high number or percentage, or both, of students enrolled or accepted for enrollment at the applicant institution who meet the eligibility requirements of Sec. 646.3;
Score: _____

(continued)

FIGURE 17.1. Technical Review Form (Student Support Services). This is the form that the reader uses to score each of the proposals before submission. The explanations included are from the selection criteria that the proposal writer should also follow so that each section is clearly identified and the reader is scoring the section as the writer intended and the proposal required.

(2) (8 points) The academic and other problems that eligible students encounter at the applicant institution; and

Score: _____

(3) (8 points) The differences between eligible Student Support Services students compared to an appropriate group, based on the following indicators:
 (i) Retention and graduation rates.
 (ii) Grade point averages.
 (iii) Graduate and professional school enrollment rates (four-year colleges only).
 (iv) Transfer rates from two-year to four-year institutions (two-year colleges only).

Total Points Assigned for Need (1-3)
Max Points (24)
Score: _____

OBJECTIVES: (8 points) [Section 646.21(b)]
The Secretary evaluates the quality of the applicant's proposed project objectives on the basis of the extent to which they are both ambitious, as related to the need data provided under paragraph (a) of this section, and attainable, given the project's plan of operation, budget, and other resources.

A1. (3 points) Persistence Rate (2-year): _____% of all participants served in the reporting year by the Student Support Services (SSS) project will persist from one academic year to the beginning of the next academic year or earn an associate degree or certificate at the grantee institution and/or transfer from a 2-year to a 4-year institution by the fall term of the next academic year.
A2. (3 points) Persistence Rate (4-year): _____% of all participants served by the SSS project will persist from one academic year to the beginning of the next academic year or will have earned a bachelor's degree at the grantee institution during the academic year.
B. (2 points) Good Academic Standing Rate (both 2- and 4-year): _____% of all enrolled participants served will meet the performance level required to stay in good academic standing at the grantee institution.
C1. Graduation and Transfer Rates (2-year):
(1 point) _____% of new participants served each year will graduate from the grantee institution with an associate degree or certificate within four (4) years,
AND
(2 points) _____% of new participants served each year will receive an associate degree or certificate from the grantee institution *and* transfer to a four-year institution within four (4) years.
C2. Graduation Rate (4-year):
(3 points) _____% of new participants served each year will graduate from the grantee institution with a bachelor's degree or equivalent within six (6) years.

Total Points Assigned for Objectives
Max Points (8)
Score: _____

(b) PLAN OF OPERATION: (30 points) [Section 646.21(c)]
The Secretary evaluates the quality of the applicant's plan of operation on the basis of the following:

(1) (3 points) The plan to inform the institutional community (students, faculty, and staff) of the goals, objectives, and services of the project and the eligibility requirements for participation in the project.

Score: _____

(2) (3 points) The plan to identify, select, and retain project participants with academic need.

Score: _____

(3) (4 points) The plan for assessing each individual participant's need for specific services and monitoring his or her academic progress at the institution to ensure satisfactory academic progress.

Score: _____

(continued)

FIGURE 17.1. *(continued)*

(4) (10 points) The plan to provide services that address the goals and objectives of the project.

Score: _____

(5) (10 points) The applicant's plan to ensure proper and efficient administration of the project, including the organizational placement of the project; the time commitment of key project staff; the specific plans for financial management, student records management, and personnel management; and, where appropriate, its plan for coordination with other programs for disadvantaged students.

Score: _____

Total Points Assigned for Plan of Operation (1-5)

Max Points (30)

Score: _____

(c) <u>INSTITUTIONAL COMMITMENT:</u> (16 points) [Section 646.21(d)]

The Secretary evaluates the institutional commitment to the proposed project on the basis of the extent to which the applicant has:

(1) (6 points) Committed facilities, equipment, supplies, personnel, and other resources to supplement the grant and enhance project services;

Score: _____

(2) (6 points) Established administrative and academic policies that enhance participants' retention at the institution and improve their chances of graduating from the institution;

Score: _____

(3) (2 points) Demonstrated a commitment to minimize the dependence on student loans in developing financial aid packages for project participants by committing institutional resources to the extent possible; and

Score: _____

(4) (2 points) Assured the full cooperation and support of the admissions, student aid, registrar and data collection and analysis components of the institution.

Score: _____

Total Points Assigned for Institutional Commitment (1-4)

Max points (16)

Score: _____

(d) <u>QUALITY OF PERSONNEL:</u> (9 points) [Section 646.21(e)]

To determine the quality of personnel the applicant plans to use, the Secretary looks for information that shows:

(1) (3 points) The qualifications required of the project director, including formal education and training in fields related to the objectives in the project, and experience in designing, managing, or implementing Student Support Services or similar projects;

Score: _____

(2) (3 points) The qualifications of other personnel to be used in the projects, including formal education, training, and work experience in fields related to the objectives of the project; and

Score: _____

(3) (3 points) The quality of the applicant's plan for employing personnel who have succeeded in overcoming barriers similar to those confronting the project's target population.

Score: _____

Total Points Assigned for Quality of Personnel (1-3)

Max Points (9)

Score: _____

(continued)

FIGURE 17.1. *(continued)*

(e) <u>BUDGET:</u> (5 points) [Section 646.21(f)]
The Secretary evaluates the extent to which the project budget is reasonable, cost-effective, and adequate to support the project.

Score: _____
Total Points Assigned for Budget
Max Points (5)
Score: _____

(f) <u>EVALUATION PLAN:</u> (8 points) [Section 646.21(g)]
The Secretary evaluates the quality of the evaluation plan for the project on the basis of the extent to which:

(1) The applicant's methods for evaluation:
   (i) (2 points) Are appropriate to the project and include both quantitative and qualitative evaluation measures; and

Score: _____
   (ii) (2 points) Examine in specific and measurable ways, using appropriate baseline data, the success of the project in improving academic achievement, retention and graduation of project participants.

Score: _____

(2) (4 points) The applicant intends to use the results of an evaluation to make programmatic changes based upon the results of project evaluation.

Score: _____
Total Points Assigned for Evaluation Plan (1-2)|
Max Points (8)
Score: _____

Status:

FIGURE 17.1. *(continued)*

Technical Review Cover Sheet				
Application	Research Foundation of CUNY on behalf of Lehman College (P042A150967)			
Selection Criteria			Points Possible	Points Scored
Need			24	24
Objectives			8	8
Plan of Operation			30	30
Institutional Commitment			16	16
Quality of Personnel			9	9
Budget			5	5
Evaluation			8	8
Competitive Priorities	1a		1	1
	1b		2	2
	2a		1	1
	2b		2	2
Totals			106	106

(continued)

FIGURE 17.2. Completed Technical Review Form (Student Support Services).

Technical Review Form

Panel #139 - FY 2015 SSS - 139: 84.042A
Research Foundation of CUNY on behalf of Lehman College (P042A150967)

NEED: Evaluate the need for a Student Support Services project proposed at the applicant institution on the basis of the extent to which the application contains clear evidence of:

1. **A high number or percentage, or both, of students enrolled or accepted for enrollment at the applicant institution who meet the eligibility requirements of §646.3;**

    Strengths:
    The applicant makes a compelling argument for the SSS program by providing statistical data show that a high number or percentage, or both, of students enrolled or accepted for enrollment. The applicant states that in 2014 total enrollment was 10,098 and of that number: 8,583 or 85% were low income; 7,675 or 76% were first generation; 7,068 or 70% were low income and first generation; 405 or 4% were students with disabilities; and 310 or 3% were both low income and disabled. The total number of students qualified to receive support was 8,482 or 84% and clearly demonstrates the need for this program.

    Weaknesses:
    No weakness noted.

    Reader's Score: 8

2. **The academic and other problems that eligible students encounter at the applicant institution; and**

    Strengths:
    The applicant clearly describes academic and other problems facing its target SSS-eligible students that keep them from obtaining a college education. Some of them are academic in nature, such as being academically unprepared for college work; failing to score sufficiently on college admission tests; and requiring improvement in English comprehension. There are also nonacademic factors such as low cognitive skills and few, if any, family role models. Students also could not understand the connection between college and career and did not perceive their need for family and other support.

    Weaknesses:
    No weakness noted.

    Reader's Score: 8

3. **The differences between eligible Student Support Services students compared to an appropriate group, based on the following indicators:**
    (i) **Retention and graduation rates.**
    (ii) **Grade-point averages.**
    (iii) **Graduate and professional school enrollment rates (four-year colleges only).**
    (iv) **Transfer rates from two-year to four-year institutions (two-year colleges only).**

    Strengths:
    (i) The applicant provided a comparison of retention rates (2013) for SSS eligible students (70%) compared to ineligible students (74%). Graduation rates (6-year cohort 2007–2013) for SSS-eligible students is 25% compared to ineligible students (34%).
    (ii) The applicant provides comparative data regarding GPAs (2012) for SSS-eligible students (2.28) compared to SSS-ineligible students (2.88).
    (iii) The applicant provides comparative data regarding graduation and professional school enrollment (2013) for SSS-eligible students (13%) compare to SSS-ineligible students (25%).
    (iv) N/A

(continued)

FIGURE 17.2. *(continued)*

207

Weaknesses:
  (i) No weakness noted.
  (ii) No weakness noted.
  (iii) No weakness noted.
  (iv) N/A

Reader's Score: 8

Reader's Total Score: 24

OBJECTIVES: Evaluate the quality of the applicant's proposed project objectives on the basis of the extent to which they are ambitious and attainable.

1.

2-Year Institutions:
% of all participants served in the reporting year by the SSS project will persist from one academic year to the beginning of the next academic year or earn an associate degree or certificate at the applicant institution and/or transfer from a 2-year to a 4-year institution by the fall term of the next academic year.

OR

4-Year Institutions:
% of all participants served by the SSS project will persist from one academic year to the beginning of the next academic year or will have earned a bachelor's degree at the applicant institution during the academic year.

Strengths:
The applicant is proposing that 85% of eligible students served will persist from one year to the next compared to the current rate of 70% of its SSS-eligible students who persist. This objective is ambitious based on need and is attainable because of the support services that will be provided, including community connections; academic support; group study sessions; cultural activities; retreats; and connections to college personnel and faculty.

Weaknesses:
No weakness noted.

Reader's Score: 3

2.

2-Year Institutions:
% of all enrolled SSS participants served will meet the performance level required to stay in good academic standing at the applicant institution.

OR

4-Year Institutions:
Good Academic Standing Rate:
% of all enrolled SSS participants served will meet the performance level required to stay in good academic standing at the applicant institution.

Strengths:
The applicant proposes that 75% of all enrolled SSS participants served will meet the performance level required to stay in good academic standing at the grantee institution. Currently 63% of SSS-eligible students are in good academic standing. This objective is ambitious and is attainable because of the proposed support services: supplemental instruction; scheduled and required group review study sessions;, intrusive advising; instructor assessments within 3 weeks of the start of each semester; academic center workshops designed to meet SSS/CIT participant academic needs; library/information literacy/research workshops; and counselor advocate regular meetings with individuals and with small groups of students.

(continued)

FIGURE 17.2. *(continued)*

Weaknesses:
No weakness noted.

Reader's Score: 2

3.

2-Year Institutions:
% of new participants served each year will graduate from the applicant institution with an associate degree or certificate within four (4) years;
(1 point) AND
% of new participants served each year will receive an associate degree or certificate from the applicant institution and transfer to a 4-year institution within 4 years.
(2 points)

OR

4-Year Institutions:
% of new participants served each year will graduate from the applicant institution with a bachelor's degree or equivalent within 6 years;
(3 points)

Strengths
The applicant is proposing 50% of SSS-eligible students served will graduate from the institution with a bachelor's degree within 6 years, compared to the current rate for SSS-eligible students of 30%. This objective is ambitious based on the identified need and attainable because of the proposed support services: creation of academic study plans; intrusive advising by the project director and dedicated counselor advocates; academic assistance when needed; early alert system; and participant progress reviews five times per year.

Weaknesses:
No weakness noted.

Reader's Score: 3

Reader's Total Score: 8

PLAN OF OPERATION: Evaluate the quality of the applicant's plan of operation on the basis of the following:

1. **The plan to inform the institutional community (students, faculty, and staff) of the goals, objectives, and services of the project and the eligibility requirements for participation in the project.**

Strengths:
The applicant provides a comprehensive plan to inform the institutional community (students, faculty, and staff) of the goals and objectives of its program. The applicant describes each activity in this segment of its plan and who is involved in administering the distribution of the information as well as the method used to disseminate the information. For example, the Principal Investigator and Project Director will collaborate with the Enrollment Management Council, Student Affairs Council, Admissions Office, Media Relations, Information Technology Center, and Telephone Manager to plan and implement a campus marketing plan and media blitz. The applicant will use a similar strategy to inform the students.

Reader's Score: 3

2. **The plan to identify, select, and retain project participants with academic need.**

Strengths:
The applicant provided a complete plan to identify, select, and retain participants with academic need. The applicant's plan is to identify more than 400 students who enter Lehman as first-time freshmen each year and who are eligible for Student Support Services (first-generation college students and/or from low-income families and/or disabled). The Program Director and/or counselor

(continued)

FIGURE 17.2. *(continued)*

will identify student need based on information contained in each program participant's application packet. The applicant will select 40 students from each freshman class in years 1 through 5. In year 1, however, they will also admit 50 sophomores and 50 juniors to the program (beginning on July 1, 90 days before the start date as permitted) for a total program enrollment of 140. The selection process also includes a point ranking system with each eligible criterion and identified need carrying a point weight. The applicant's plan to retain students is also thorough, as it contains the required support services that promote academic achievement, including tutoring and mentoring.

Weaknesses:
No weakness noted.

Reader's Score: 3

3. **The plan for assessing each individual participant's need for specific services and monitoring his or her academic progress at the institution to ensure satisfactory academic progress.**

Strengths:
The applicant provides a clear plan to assess specific individual needs and monitor academic progress, beginning with each student completing a pre-selection needs assessment that includes high school and/or previous college GPA; ACT or SAT test scores; regents test results in Science, Mathematics, Global Studies, American History and English; and a composite admissions score. This is administered through a system called Cooperative Institutional Research Profile (CIRP). Once the student is admitted into the program, they complete a computerized Discover® Profile at the Career Services Center, a Holland Type Profile within Discover. An educational plan is then developed specifically to meet the student's identified needs as well as program goals and objectives. Students are monitored through progress reports available within the first 3 weeks of the semester. A follow-up process is also described.

Weaknesses:
No weakness noted.

Reader's Score: 4

4. **The plan to provide services that address the goals and objectives of the project.**

Strengths:
The applicant clearly describes its plan to provide required and permissible services that address the goals and objectives of the program: improving retention, increasing GPAs, and improving graduation rates. The applicant provides a comprehensive list of required and permissible services that will be provided to the program participants while identifying the staff involved in each activity.

Reader's Score: 10

5. **The applicant's plan to ensure proper and efficient administration of the project, including the organizational placement of the project; the time commitment of key project staff; the specific plans for financial management, student records management, and personnel management; and, where appropriate, its plan for coordination with other programs for disadvantaged students.**

Strengths:
The applicant describes in detail its commitment to ensure the effective and efficient administration of the project as described in its organizational chart and placement of key personnel. The applicant states that the Project Director is responsible for the day-to-day oversight of the SSS program and reports to the Principal Investigator. The applicant also indicates that the Director will collaborate with other Lehman Academic and Student Services Offices to assure efficient and effective management of the project and will be a member of the Enrollment Management Council that meets weekly and is chaired by the Associate Provost. The applicant also presents the time commitment for project staff and provides a timeline of activities and indicates the responsible staff. The applicant describes records management—for example, student records are

(continued)

FIGURE 17.2. *(continued)*

210

kept electronically and in paper format. The applicant describes its coordination of services with organizations and agencies.

Weaknesses:
No weakness noted.

Reader's Score: 10

Reader's Total Score: 30

INSTITUTIONAL COMMITMENT: Evaluate the quality of the applicant's institutional commitment, extent to which the applicant has:

1. **Committed facilities, equipment, supplies, personnel, and other resources to supplement the grant and enhance project services;**

   Strengths:
   The applicant describes its commitment to the SSS program by describing the facility, its location, and equipment and supplies to be used in support of the SSS program. For example, the program office will be located in a renovated space in the "Old Gym" in the center of the campus that is readily accessible to all. The thoroughness with which the applicant describes each allocated resource demonstrates its commitment to the success of the project—for example, the allocated space and hours of operation for the Information Technology center and the allocation of adjunct staff for tutoring.

   Reader's Score: 6

2. **Established administrative and academic policies that enhance participants' retention at the institution and improve their chances of graduating from the institution;**

   Strengths:
   The applicant details administrative and academic policy designed to enhance retention and graduation. For example, the applicant's staff will be represented on the Enrollment Management Council which monitors admission and retention of students; the Student Affairs Council which monitors registration, campus activities, clubs, career services, and counseling, and on the appeals committee which reviews student requests for probation. Also, the applicant conducts a Student Experience Survey that identifies students with good grades who are at risk of leaving. The applicant also monitors student grades to determine if they are at risk of falling below a 2.0 and, if necessary initiates corrective action.

   Weaknesses:
   No weakness noted.

   Reader's Score: 6

3. **Demonstrated a commitment to minimize the dependence on student loans in developing financial aid packages for project participants by committing institutional resources to the extent possible; and**

   Strengths:
   The applicant clearly demonstrates its commitment to minimize student loan dependency as evidenced by the applicant's establishment of a scholarship endowment of $1 million and its quest to raise $1 billion to assure that students continue to have a low borrowing rate as 80% of its students are Pell grant recipients. To further demonstrate its commitment to minimize student loan dependency the applicant waives a total of four 3-credit courses for SSS/CIT participants to reduce their reliance on financial aid and so that students can maintain the 15 credits per semester and 30 credits per year levels needed to graduate in 4 years. At a cost of $200/credit this is a total of $280,000 for each student cohort. This is enabled because SSS/CIT funding pays the cost of instruction at a total of $20,000/year for each cohort.

   Weaknesses:
   No weakness noted.

   Reader's Score: 2

(continued)

FIGURE 17.2. *(continued)*

4. **Assured the full cooperation and support of the admissions, student aid, registrar, and data collection and analysis components of the institution.**

Strengths:
The applicant clearly describes the full cooperation and support of the admissions, student aid, registrar, and data collection analysis departments. The program collaborates with the Enrollment Management Council consisting of Directors of Admissions, Testing, Academic Advisement, Institutional Research, SEEK, Freshman Year Initiative, Academic Support Excellence, School/College Collaboratives. and College Now. The SSS/CIT Director also serves on the Student Affairs Council, chaired by the Vice President of Student Affairs. More important, the Vice President of Student Affairs and the Associate Provost for Enrollment Management are part of the President's Cabinet and meet regularly with the Vice Presidents of Administration, Institutional Advancement, Institutional Research, and Academic Affairs to review general and critical items and programs. The Dean of Education meets regularly with the Dean's Council of the College. The President of the College has made a firm commitment to fully support this Project.

Weaknesses:
No weakness noted.

Reader's Score: 2

Reader's Total Score: 16

QUALITY OF PERSONNEL: To determine the quality of personnel the applicant plans to use, the Secretary looks for information that shows:

1. **The qualifications required of the project director, including formal education and training in fields related to the objectives of the project, and experience in designing, managing, or implementing Student Support Services or similar projects;**

Strengths:
The applicant states that the required qualification, education, and training for its Project Director is a master's degree in education, administration, counseling, or a related field; 3 to 5 years of increasingly responsible administrative experience in an equal educational opportunity setting in higher education; 5 years of experience working with first-generation, low-income, and disabled students in higher education; and demonstrated experience in project management for higher education programs. Also, the Director is expected to demonstrate expertise in all aspects of program administration: personnel supervision; developing and monitoring budgets; writing program reports; and conducting program evaluation. The Director must have demonstrated the ability to work with faculty, administrators, campus officials, community agencies, and schools and students from diverse backgrounds. A personal background similar to the target population is preferred. The Director will allocate 50% time to the project.

Weaknesses:
No weakness noted.

Reader's Score: 3

2. **The qualifications required of other personnel to be used in the project, including formal education, training, and work experience in fields related to the objectives of the project; and**

Strengths:
The applicant distinctly describes the required qualifications, education, and training required for other key personnel. For example, the Academic Counselor Advocates preferably have a master's degree in education, administration, counseling or a related field; 3 to 5 years of increasingly responsible experience in career planning, counseling, group facilitation, leadership training, academic advisement, workshop planning and delivery; demonstrated ability to work with diverse college students; ability to work a flexible schedule including nights and weekends as necessary; excellent organization, writing and oral communication skills; and a background similar to the target population.

(continued)

FIGURE 17.2. *(continued)*

Weaknesses:
No weakness noted.

Reader's Score: 3

3. **The quality of the applicant's plan for employing personnel who have succeeded in overcoming barriers similar to those confronting the project's target population.**

Strengths:
The applicant thoroughly describes its plan to hire individuals who have overcome similar barriers by widely distributing position openings to TRIO alumni (through long-standing programs) and emails to established programs which contain links to the job posting on the applicant's website. Applicant will also place job vacancies in diverse group publications so as to attract a diverse pool of applicants.

Weaknesses:
No weakness noted.

Reader's Score: 3

Reader's Total Score: 9

BUDGET: Evaluate the extent to which the project budget is reasonable, cost-effective, and adequate to support the project.

Strengths:
Applicant's budget is cost-effective, efficient and reasonable given that they are purposing to serve 140 students at a total cost of $217,475. Applicant's line items align with budget narrative.

Weaknesses:
No weakness noted.

Reader's Total Score: 5

EVALUATION PLAN: Evaluate the quality of the evaluation plan for the project on the basis of the extent to which:

1. **The applicant's methods for evaluation are appropriate to the project and include both quantitative and qualitative evaluation measures;**

Strengths:
The applicant provides a clear evaluation plan that consists of quantifiable (quantitative and qualitative) data that measures the program progress toward meeting stated goals and objectives and assesses the overall effectiveness of the program. The applicant's use of quantifiable data also provides valuable information for the formative and summative components of the evaluation.

Weaknesses:
No weakness noted.

Reader's Score: 2

2. **The applicant's methods for evaluation examine in specific and measurable ways, using appropriate baseline data, the success of the project in improving academic achievement, retention and graduation of project participants; and**

Strengths:
The applicant clearly describes its evaluation plan and uses quantitative and qualitative baseline data in measurable ways that are objective driven to determine if stated objectives are being met. For example, the applicant's objective for a 50% increase in graduation is measured by the extent to which the services provided can be linked to the project's success in achieving the objective.

Weaknesses:
No weakness noted.

Reader's Score: 2

(continued)

FIGURE 17.2. *(continued)*

3. **The applicant intends to use the results of an evaluation to make programmatic changes based upon the results of project evaluation.**

   Strengths:
   The applicant provides a sound formative and summative evaluation plan designed to determine what programmatic changes are needed, and to assess the overall impact the program has on program participants. To determine the overall outcome and program impact the applicant will use the Blumen database, the College Business Intelligence System, and annual Student Experience Surveys, as well as exit surveys from counselor advocate/participant advisory meetings and workshops at least eight times per semester to collect a wide range of data on each participant. This data collection strategy is designed to provide accurate and valuable information about the program's success in meeting the needs of the students.

   Weaknesses:
   No weakness noted.

   Reader's Score: 4

Reader's Total Score: 8

PRIORITY QUESTIONS
Competitive Preference Priority 1(a)
Influencing the Development of Non-Cognitive Factors. The Department is using this competitive preference priority to focus on postsecondary persistence and completion rates among high-need students. Postsecondary completion rates among students from high-need backgrounds are unacceptably low. The Department believes that SSS projects can play a strong role in improving postsecondary outcomes by placing a greater emphasis on strategies designed to influence the development of non-cognitive skills. Evaluate the quality of the applicant's strategy to develop the non-cognitive skills of students.

   Strengths:
   The applicant addresses this priority by designing a program that assures continuing attention to and development of students' non-cognitive skills, shown to be critical to college, career, and life success. This strategy is based on suggestions that non-cognitive factors can play an important role in students' academic, career, and life outcomes (Walton & Cohen, 2011; Stephens, Hamedani, & Destin, 2014). Non-cognitive skills encompass a broad range of behaviors, strategies, and attitudes: "academic behaviors (including attendance and homework completion), academic mindsets (including a sense of belonging in the academic community and believing that academic achievement improves with effort), perseverance (including tenacity and self-discipline), social and emotional skills (including cooperation, empathy, and adaptability), and approaches toward learning strategies (such as executive functions, attention, goal-setting, curiosity, problem solving, self-regulating learning, study skills, and the ability to work cooperatively with others)."

   (SSS RFP 2015). The study proved to be effective and to have a positive effect on the students.

   Weaknesses:
   No weakness noted.

   Reader's Score: 1

(continued)

FIGURE 17.2. *(continued)*

Competitive Preference Priority 1(b)

Non-Cognitive Factors Supported by Moderate Evidence of Effectiveness. In recent years, the Department has placed an increasing emphasis on promoting evidence-based practices through our grant competitions. We believe that encouraging applicants to focus on proven strategies can only enhance the quality of our competitions. Accordingly, within the competitive priority for influencing the development of non-cognitive factors—Competitive Preference Priority 1(a)—we give additional competitive preference to applications that submit moderate evidence of effectiveness that supports their proposed strategy for addressing non-cognitive factors. The Secretary may award 2 points for this Priority depending upon how well the applicant addresses the moderate evidence of effectiveness that supports their proposed strategy. Evaluate the relevance of the moderate evidence of effectiveness submitted by the applicant.

Strengths:
The applicant uses moderate evidence of effectiveness by citing the research study done by Stephens, Hamedani, & Destin (2014),y which is relevant to the applicant's project for the following reasons: applicant's students are non-traditional students who have enrolled at the institution as first-time full-time freshman or transfer students with 15 to 45 credits and are, for the most part, first-generation, low-income students (80%): the urban environments in which they reside and the high schools they attend are, for the most part, populated with people like themselves; and few of applicant's students had experience in a diverse setting and so the institution is their first encounter with diversity. Stephens et al. (2014) presented evidence from a randomized controlled study that used a difference-education intervention with incoming students that was "designed to demonstrate to incoming students how their diverse backgrounds can shape what they experience in college." The intervention strategy worked because when the social class achievement gap was eliminated the students tend to seek our professors for classwork clarification.

Weaknesses:
No weakness noted.

Reader's Score: 2

Competitive Preference Priority 2(a)

Providing Individualized Counseling for Personal, Career, and Academic Matters. The Department is using this Competitive Preference Priority to focus on improved individualized counseling to students. The Department believes that SSS projects can play a strong role in improving postsecondary outcomes by placing a greater emphasis on proactive coaching strategies designed to increase student success. Evaluate the quality of the applicant's strategy to provide individualized counseling to students for personal, career, and academic matters.

Strengths:
The applicant describes its strategy to address Individualized Counseling for personal, career, and academic matters. The applicant cites the Bettinger and Baker (2011) study, which is relevant to the project because of the nature of its student population the applicant is proposing to serve. Study participants were first-time full-time freshman or transfer students with 15 to 45 credits and were, for the most part, first-generation, low-income students (80%). The urban high schools they graduated from did a poor job of preparing them for college and too many lacked the skills they need to make appropriate choices on their own. Therefore, the need for individualized counseling proved to be central to the success of the students' educational achievement. Therefore, the project's individualized counseling strategy employs an Intrusive Advisement Model and is implemented by one full-time and one part-time counselor advocate. Although the project does not employ an external provider such as InsideTrack (Bettinger & Baker, 2011), its strategies for maintaining ongoing, intrusive contact with students use email, text, and phone to reach out to students at least once a week. According to the study this strategy proved to be beneficial to the students.

(continued)

FIGURE 17.2. *(continued)*

Weaknesses:
No weakness noted.

Reader's Score: 1

Competitive Preference Priority 2(b)

Individual Counseling Activities Based on Moderate Evidence of Effectiveness. This competitive preference priority invites applicants to propose ways to improve the effectiveness of counseling using evidence-based practices, which could include coaching or other strategies. Accordingly, within the competitive priority for individualized counseling, we give additional competitive preference to applications that submit moderate evidence of effectiveness that supports their proposed strategies for providing individualized counseling. The Secretary may award 2 points for this Priority depending upon how well the applicant addresses the moderate evidence of effectiveness that supports their proposed strategy. Evaluate the relevance of the moderate evidence of effectiveness submitted by the applicant.

Strengths:
The applicant's strategy for addressing individualized counseling is based moderate evidence of effectiveness from the research study reported by Bettinger and Baker (2011). They also make the point, in their review of the literature, that educational interventions have attempted to use college counseling models to improve college outcomes. These treatments, "identified as 'counseling' or 'advising' vary greatly—some are strictly academic, others focus on study skills and social needs. The applicant's Intrusive Advising Model has a very clear process that all counselor advocates follow, including: individual check sheets and protocols individualized for each student; semester transcripts, sample course papers, test grades, and academic support usage. In addition counselor advocates use the college Long Range Academic Planning web-based tool to assure that students are progressing on a regular basis and can work with the student to modify, accelerate, or decelerate progress toward graduation.

Weaknesses: No weakness noted.

Reader's Score: 2

FIGURE 17.2. *(continued)*

CHAPTER 18

Next Steps

So you have reached the last chapter and have tried some of the Practice Exercises at the end of the book. Maybe you have submitted your proposal and are waiting to hear the funder's decision. Where should you go from here to hone your skills and produce winning proposals? **My suggestion is that you start over and develop another grant proposal.** It often takes 6 months or more to get a decision on the status of your proposal. With federal grants, where the fiscal year begins on October 1, you will often have to wait until mid-September for notification of funding. Notification on continuing grants sometimes comes in August so nonfunded programs that have had funding for the last project period can prepare for the shutdown process before the fall semester starts.

Frequent practice in the process of creating a winning proposal is the best way to become proficient. In addition, engagement with the individuals at your institution/organization who are there to assist you can be more helpful as you get to know them. If the ORSP offers workshops, you should definitely participate. Now that you have developed a grant proposal, their suggestions and techniques will make a lot more sense to you.

There are also some other do-ahead activities that will prepare you for future proposals.

1. *Get to know the individuals at your institution/organization who are the go-to people for critical information and statistics you will need to obtain for your proposals.*

   Why?

   - It is critical to establish and maintain relationships with individuals who are in a position to help you get the accurate and up-to-date information needed to complete your proposals—usually these are the individuals in institutional research.

- When you discuss the types of information you may need, they may be able to design a query that can be run against institutional data when you need it.

- This will reduce the effort needed to generate the data you need and will speed the process of getting the information.

2. *Visit your institutional ORSP **early and often** as you develop a proposal and as you draft the first sections and especially the budget. Also send them a copy of the RFP via e-mail so they can review it and assist you in assuring that you respond accurately and fully to the proposal requirements.*

   Why?

   - Those who work in the ORSP are the most experienced individuals on your campus to:
     - Review RFP specifications.
     - Highlight the nuances that those new to the proposal process might miss when interpreting and following budget guidelines.
     - Have the most up-to-date information on fringe and indirect rates.
     - Know which expenses are allowable and which are unallowable.
     - Understand the requirements and the process for uploading your proposal.
     - Submit the proposal.

3. *Get on mailing lists for corporate, foundation, and government funders in order to receive timely notification of upcoming competitions or solicitations and regularly search funding sites. If your institution/organization has a subscription to PIVOT (**https://pivot.cos.com**), you can enter key search terms and get a regular summary of new opportunities e-mailed to you. Check the USDE Forecast of Funding Opportunities at **www2.ed.gov/fund/grant/find/edlite-forecast.html?src=ft**. Consult the Federal Register. Ask your OSRP to provide notice of RFPs in your areas of interest when they hear about them.*

   Why?

   - To have early awareness of upcoming opportunities.

   - So you have time to begin the process of determining if the opportunity fits your institution/organization and begin preparing your proposal.

   - To learn which RFPs are cyclical, that is, they are available each year, every 3 years, or every 5 years.

   - For cyclical RFPs you can begin to plan for the next competition well in advance of the announcement.

   - The Federal Register often published notifications of funding being considered by Congress and before they are officially released.

4. *Take advantage of all opportunities to attend workshops and webinars on preparing proposals for the funders you are likely to approach with a proposal.*

   Why?

   - Workshops and webinars conducted by support organizations, like the Council for Educational Opportunity, use specific examples and interpret the guidelines in a systematic fashion.

   - If your institution is a member of certain organizations, the workshops are free and are offered in several locations around the United States and in Puerto Rico in years when grants are offered.

   - These organizations will read part of your proposal and offer constructive feedback if you bring a section to the workshop. As the need and Plan of Operation sections are worth the most points, 24 and 30 respectively, these are probably what you should submit for comment.

5. *Maintain a current "needs" section for use in a variety of proposals and update it, perhaps once a year to reflect changes.*

   Why?

   - Most RFPs want you to provide an assessment of need for your institution/organization, the individuals you intend to serve, and the community where they and your institution/organization are located, with evidence culled from published sources.

   - Information from American FactFinder changes yearly and regular updating of community demographics saves time. (**https://factfinder.census.gov/faces/nav/jsf/pages/index.xhtml**)

   - Maintaining such a section alleviates some of the work required to formulate a recent profile and saves the time spent reviewing all of the sources essential to create a comprehensive profile.

   - The section can easily be reviewed and updated for various proposals.

6. *Create a database of institutional data and academic statistics that is updated yearly with information on demographics, graduation rates, progress toward graduation, retention, persistence, GPAs, and DFWI (D or F grades, Withdrawals and Incomplete grades in gateway courses) and update it once a year to reflect changes.*

   Why?

   - The RFP will require you to indicate the current state of the needs you highlight in your proposal.

   - In order to determine the percentages to assign to project objectives you need to know your current situation so that your outcomes will be realistic and attainable but ambitious.

   - You can avoid a last-minute rush situation that will put pressure on you and on your institutional research department.

7. *Through contact with your ORSP, maintain current information on requirements for budgeting and institutional/organizational approvals, deadlines for submission to the office, and internal systems for creating proposals. Also let the office know as soon as you even think that you will be submitting a proposal for an upcoming competition.*

   Why?

   - Budget requirements can change if fringe rates are adjusted.
   - Indirect cost percentages are subject to revision.
   - Internal systems may be updated and deadlines can change due to the number of anticipated proposals.
   - The sooner they know that you are planning to submit, the better they can assist you.

8. *Go to funder websites and read abstracts of proposals that have been funded within the past 2 or 3 years to see the types of activities, ideas, and programs they fund. Visit the websites created by programs that have been funded to determine goals, objectives, and activities they implement and how they evaluate their program accomplishments.*

   Why?

   - Get an idea of the types of projects that have been funded.
   - Get ideas for your proposal or project.
   - Determine if your ideas either fit or do not fit the funding profile.
   - Learn as much as you can about the funder.

9. *Subscribe to the IES mailing list (***www.ies.ed.gov***).*

   Why?

   - The IES frequently publishes the results of its reviews of research findings in education. You will get a notification and summary of each review they publish and/or new publications based on summaries of research.
   - Summaries are very helpful as alerts to what is happening in educational research.
   - You will gain information on effective practices in teaching and learning.
   - These are the studies that you will use in invitational or competitive priorities.

10. *Sign up to become a peer reviewer for education grant competitions (***www2.ed.gov/about/offices/list/ope/peer-reviewers/index.html***).*

    Why?

    - This is an excellent professional development opportunity
    - It's a chance to serve the education community.

- To obtain training and preparation, as well as benefit from individual support for each review.
- To learn about new and innovative ideas in your field.
- To engage in the grant-making process while meeting and networking with other experts in your profession.
- To get an in-depth look at the effort involved in the grant evaluation process.
- To gain perspective and skills that are applicable in other professional endeavors.

11. *Participate in campus meetings about initiatives and assessment of current practice and read any strategic planning documents that are available.*

    Why?

    - To learn about the student experience on campus.
    - So you can understand the student support services being implemented or those that are needed.
    - To become familiar with professional development efforts on campus.
    - To gain insight into the innovative approaches your colleagues are initiating.
    - To understand the institutional vision and mission and become informed about short- and long-range goals.
    - Learn about colleagues or administrators who might be interested in pursuing institutional RFPs.

12. *Develop expertise about program evaluation by using resources pertaining to qualitative and quantitative evaluation/research methods.*

    Why?

    - The evaluation is frequently the last and most poorly written section of the proposal.
    - Evaluation is critical to showing how you will know that you have achieved your goals and objectives.
    - To choose the right evaluation for your project methods.
    - To identify appropriate assessment tools and use the best and most suitable analysis methods.
    - To discuss evaluation intelligently with an outside evaluator if you use one.
    - To identify the information you need from the college office of institutional research.
    - To understand the strengths and weaknesses of different evaluation strategies.

- Review one of the following websites:
  - **https://innovation.ed.gov/what-we-do/teacher-quality/ supporting-effective-educator-development-grant-program/ evaluation-resources**
  - **https://ies.ed.gov/ncee/wwc/Multimedia/43**

13. *Google the phrase "common errors made in proposals" and read the entries that come up to determine the most frequent errors that submitters make. You and at least one other person should check and recheck the proposal before final submission.*

    Why?

    - Many proposals are not forwarded to the review process at all because of small mistakes that might have been avoided.
    - Familiarity with the proposal may lead to seeing connections that really aren't explicit.
    - Even if numbering is turned on the word processing program only does what you tell it.
    - Your proposal may not be read if you have any formatting errors.

14. *Use the web resources in Appendix B to further review how to successfully respond to RFPs or to various selection criteria within the RFP before or during your proposal-writing process.*

    Why?

    - The web resources that are provided in Appendix B have been carefully reviewed and selected.
    - They provide additional information and assistance to be used before or during the proposal-writing process.

Why Invest Your Time and Effort?

By far the most important reason to invest time and effort in grant writing is to help underserved students in your communities close the academic achievement gap that, despite our best efforts, keeps widening. When I first began writing proposals there was one project that I really wanted to have funded. I approached a colleague, Eileen Allman, and she worked with me to create a paragraph that I still use in various forms today because it encapsulates why I continue to write proposals after 36 years.

> Urban schools will be large and troubled for the foreseeable future. Ways must be found to create internal and external environments in which students can flourish. Through [name of program] we are determined to create those settings and engage school and community members to support student success as evidenced by successful transitions through graduation from high school, college admission, and attainment of a baccalaureate degree. If any school anywhere has the resources

to accomplish, and would benefit by, a comprehensive, collaborative approach to attaining its educational objectives, [name of school] is it. [Name of school], located in one of the most blighted urban areas in the country, too easily elicits a fatalistic shrug of the shoulder. Yet, we cannot afford to lose another generation to "might have been." The future of [name of school] is the future of urban education and so the importance of this program cannot be overemphasized. We see what can be, believe that it can be done, and know that we have the power to do it.

There are also several more personal reasons why you should engage in proposal writing and work to become proficient. First, you will learn and improve a valuable skill set; second, you will have the wherewithal to respond to needs you see within your institution/organization and either take the lead or work with a group to seek the additional resources necessary; third, the process of proposal writing is akin to systematic problem solving and you will greatly improve your ability to work through complex issues and questions; you will be able to serve as a mentor and collaborator for others, including your students, who want to learn the proposal-writing process; and finally, if you have aspirations for leadership in your field, successful proposal writing is a good skill to have featured on your résumé.

Improving Data Gathering and Synthesis Skills

If you are going to write proposals on a regular basis, you want improve your skills and knowledge and become proficient. In addition, the process of writing and organizing a proposal will add to your skill set. Many sections of a proposal involve the gathering of facts and numbers and organizing them into charts and tables that show readers and funders the serious need for what you are proposing. Gathering the data and formatting charts, tables, and figures is a learned skill. The more you practice the better you will get at presenting your case. Fortunately, this skill can serve many other purposes in your work, or even community, life. If you teach, if you volunteer for community agencies, if you make a presentation to a group, if you are disseminating the findings from a project or if you are preparing an article for presentation this skill will be of great value.

Seeing the Whole Picture

The proposal, as a whole, is a systematic, relational presentation of facts and figures to demonstrate need and show how your approach to addressing it through the activities you propose (that are supported by moderate or strong evidence) will result in achieving the goals and objectives you propose and show that improvement ensues through evaluation using appropriate measures. As you write more proposals, you will find that you become more and more proficient at seeing and communicating the connections among and between goals, objectives, activities, and outcomes. This will result in improving your ability to make connections almost as second nature in your work or community life.

Gain Deep Knowledge of the Institution

You will become more astute at viewing your institution, organization, or community in terms of *possibilities*. How can small to medium changes improve student outcomes, community participation, faculty work, collaboration, and/or enthusiasm? How can student, faculty, and administrative motivation for change be kindled? What are the changes that individuals believe are needed to strengthen the institution?

Develop Leadership Skills

Your own leadership and group process skills will develop as you engage with others in identifying RFPs, developing a conceptual theme, conducting a consensus process, defining the proposal sections, establishing need, articulating goals and objectives, finding proven activities, planning the process, developing a budget, and formulating the evaluation (with or without an evaluation consultant). Perhaps the greatest leadership and group process achievement will be your management of the process from start to finish as you shepherd the proposal through the various stages of writing, reviewing, rewriting, scoring, editing, and finalizing of the version that is ultimately submitted for funding on time, on budget, with proper formatting before the deadline. You will also have the opportunity to demonstrate patience as you wait, hope, wonder, and wish to hear that you have been successful and funded!!!

Sharpen Critical Thinking Skills

The process of writing a proposal demands the ability to write succinctly, present complex ideas understandably, systematically engage in problem solving, search, synthesize, and apply research literature, establish relationships among proposal components, work through and solve complex issues and questions, create a compelling narrative, and present a coherent request in a way that will appeal to readers. While you may not possess all of these critical skills when you start on your proposal effort, you will certainly develop them in the process and will also learn from others in your group or on your team.

Better Assist Others

The knowledge and skills you develop as a proposal writer will improve your value as a mentor and collaborator for colleagues, students, and others who want to develop their proposal-writing skills. Although you already have academic skills, engaging in proposal writing, especially as part of a group, will force you to rethink, recall, and revise your early experiences in producing a complex, concise, evidence-based document using a specific format. In a way, this is a new skill for you or at least a different application of prior knowledge. The experience will enable you to identify with the problems and pitfalls students face and improve your approach to teaching, mentoring, and grading.

Practice Exercises

The practice exercises in this section will enable you to answer questions about a planned or in-process proposal. The information can be gathered with a group or by individuals within a group and then synthesized and used to create narrative text.

Abstract (Chapter 7, p. 102; Chapter 8, pp. 106–107)

This first section provides questions about the usual elements that the RFP specifies for the abstract. Once the prompts are answered a narrative can easily be written. The abstract should address five key elements about your proposal:

- *Purpose:* **Why** are you conducting this project and/or what is the purpose of the RFP; what does the funder emphasize as the purpose of the solicitation? **What** are your goals/objectives?
- *Participants:* **Whom** will you serve? **Where** will you serve them? **How** many will be participating? **What** are their needs that you will address?
- *Methods:* **What** activities, supports, materials, classes, advising will you use? **How** will you deliver the components of your project? **When** will you deliver them? **Who** will deliver them? **What** data and information will you collect?
- *Evaluation:* **What** measures will you use to assess the success in achieving each objective? **Who** will collect and analyze the data?
- *Sustainability, significance, and dissemination:* **How** will the project activities continue after funding ends? **How** will the outcomes contribute to practice? **How** will you let others know about your findings?

Column 1 in the following table names the categories for all the selection criteria in a proposal. It is suggested that you use it to outline the relevant aspects of the proposal to determine if the aspects fit together and if the relationships are obvious. Each section can be expanded to outline several needs, goals, objectives, and the associated details for Plan of Operation, administration, evaluation, budget, and dissemination. The Master Table provided in Chapter 6 is an elaborated version of the table below.

Area	
Introduction	
Need	
Goal(s)	
Objectives	
Ambitious	
Attainable	
Plan of Operation	
Notify constituencies	
Identify, select, and enroll participants	
Assessing need for services	
Plan for services	
Ensure effective administration	
Evaluation	
Budget	
Dissemination	
Significance	
Sustainability	
Invitational priorities	
Competitive priorities	
Logic model	

Introduction (Chapter 7, p. 102; Chapter 8, pp. 107–108)

1. Locate the most recent strategic plan for your institution/organization and use it to craft a compelling section highlighting strengths and weaknesses and how the strengths can be developed and the weaknesses improved to contribute to the growth of the institution and increase its success organizationally, academically, and financially.

2. Use the information from Question 1 to focus on an area of high need that will best contribute to strengthening your institution/organization and describe how improvement in this area will impact its success.

3. Identify other areas of high need within your institution/organization and answer question 2 for each area.

Statement of Need (Chapter 7, p. 102; Chapter 10)

1. Based on your answer to Question 2 above, use community data (**http://factfinder.census.gov/faces/nav/jsf/pages/index.xhtml**), your own institutional data (institutional research office or Facebook), and state and/or local data on educational achievement (college readiness, college access, standardized test scores, aspiration for higher education) to provide evidence that the area you have selected is indeed a high-need area.

2. Repeat step 1 for other areas you have identified in question 3 above.

Goals and Objectives (Chapter 7, pp. 102–103; Chapter 11)

1. Using the needs identified above, create one or more overarching goals that your proposed project will accomplish to strengthen your institution.

2. For each goal create several SMART objectives that will lead to goal achievement.

3. For each objective explain why it is ambitious but achievable using current institution/organization data (obtained in the previous section) and references to the activities described in the next section.

4. Repeat steps 1–3 for other areas of need that have been identified.

Plan of Operation (Chapter 7, p. 103; Chapter 12)

1. Create general notes for informing your constituencies that can be used for other areas you address.

2. For each area, outline how you will identify, recruit/select, and enroll participants

3. Based on participants and their possible needs, show how you will develop a profile of each participant to customize the services they will receive.

4. Based on overall needs, goals, and objectives and individual participant needs, describe in detail the services you will provide to assure achievement of your goals and objectives.

5. Create general notes on how the project will be organized for effective and efficient administration that may be applicable to other areas you address.

6. Repeat steps 1–5 for the other areas you have identified.

Evaluation (Chapter 7, pp. 103–104; Chapter 13)

1. Identify the formative/summative, process/product measures to be used to provide evidence that goals and objectives have been met.

2. Show how formative/process measures will be used to modify your project as needed to improve outcomes.

3. Suggest the ways in which data may be analyzed and define treatment of both qualitative and quantitative measures.

4. Repeat steps 1–3 for other areas.

Budget (Chapter 7, p. 105; Chapter 14)

1. Create a working budget, using a spreadsheet with formulas in Excel that can probably be used to budget each area you consider.

2. Create a sample budget narrative describing the responsibilities and compensation of each position and justification for other than personnel expenses.

Competitive Priorities (Chapter 16)

1. Using the invitational/competitive priorities presented in Table 16.1, prepare sections on one or more of your areas of need using data provided by the WWC (**http://ies.ed.gov/ncee/wwc**).

Logic Model (Chapter 9)

1. Using the information presented in Chapter 9 on developing a logic model, present a general logic model for one of the areas of need you selected in the Introduction section.

Table of Need Categories with Sorted Needs

Category 1	Category 2	Category 3	Category 4	Category 5

Forms

Summary Chart for Respondent Rankings

Each respondent ranks all the statements. The average ranking is calculated by multiplying the numbers in each cell as follows: A = $N \times 4$; B = $N \times 3$; C = $N \times 2$; D = $N \times 1$. The total of A, B, C, and D should be divided by the total number of respondents across the A to D cells.

	A	B	C	D	Average Ranking
Statement 1					
Statement 2					
Statement 3					
Statement 4					
Statement 5					
Statement 6					
Statement 7					

Forms

Summary of SWOT Components

Use one chart for each person or a large summary chart for the group. Each cell of the chart should be filled in with comments or statements relevant to Internal-Strengths; Internal-Weaknesses; External-Strengths; External-Weaknesses and how the strengths and weaknesses afford the organization opportunities or threats.

	Internal	External
Positive	**Strengths**	**Opportunities**
Negative	**Weaknesses**	**Threats**

Forms

FORM 4

Need Chart (Use with American FactFinder Data for County, City, or ZIP Code)

Subject			
	Total	Males	Females
	% Estimate	% Estimate	% Estimate
Population 25 Years and Over			
Less than 9th grade			
9th–12th grade, no diploma			
High school graduate (includes equivalency)			
Some college, no degree			
Associate degree			
Bachelor's degree			
Graduate or professional degree			
Population 25 to 34 years			
High school graduate or higher			
Bachelor's degree or higher			
Race and Hispanic or Latino Origin by Educational Attainment			
White alone, not Hispanic or Latino			
High school graduate or higher			
Bachelor's degree or higher			
Black			
High school graduate or higher			
Bachelor's degree or higher			
American Indian/Alaska Native			
High school graduate or higher			
Bachelor's degree or higher			
Asian			
High school graduate or higher			
Bachelor's degree or higher			

(continued)

Note. Margin of error = 0.1–0.2. Data from **https://factfinder.census.gov/faces/nav/jsf/pages/index.xhtml**.

Forms

	Total % Estimate	Males % Estimate	Females % Estimate
Native Hawaiian/Other Pacific Islander			
High school graduate or higher			
Bachelor's degree or higher			
Hispanic or Latino Origin			
High school graduate or higher			
Bachelor's degree or higher			
Poverty Rate			
Less than high school graduate			
High School graduate (includes equivalency)			
Some college or associate degree			
Bachelor's degree or higher			

FORM 5

Project Overview Chart

Grant	Goal	Objectives	Population	Activities	Outcomes
A					
B					
C					
D					

Master Table

Project Goal

Need	Objective	Activity	Ambitious	Attainable	Description	Output	Outcome	Evaluation	Staff	Budget

(continued)

Forms

Master Table *(page 2 of 3)*

Project Goal

Need	Objective	Activity	Ambitious	Attainable	Description	Output	Outcome	Evaluation	Staff	Budget

(continued)

Master Table *(page 3 of 3)*

Project Goal

Need	Objective	Activity	Ambitious	Attainable	Description	Output	Outcome	Evaluation	Staff	Budget

Budget Numbers and Total Budget Numbers for a Proposal with Three Programs Showing Cost Splits

	Program 1	Program 2	Program 3
Project coordinator Salary/%			
Site coordinator Salary/%			
Instructor Salary/%			
Program adviser Salary/%			
Group leader Salary/%			
Tutor Salary/%			
Other than personnel costs			
Total component cost			
Indirect costs @ _____%			
Program activity total			

Note. % = percent of time spent on activity.

Forms

Sub-Tables Created from the Master Table to Assure Content Match

Project Goal, Objective, and Evaluative Measures

Goal	Objective	Evaluative measures

Project Goal, Objective, and Activities

Goal	Objective	Activities

Project Activities, and Descriptions

Project activities	Descriptions

FORM 9

Summary of Performance Measures, Activities, and Evaluative Measures

Performance measure	Objective	Activities	Evaluative measures

Summary of Current Research on Proposal Components to be Implemented

Activity	Literature	Summary

Forms

FORM 11

Activities, Descriptions, Outputs, Outcomes, Measures, Leader

Activities	Descriptions	Outputs	Outcomes	Measures	Leader
Target Group:					

Evaluation Process and Measures for Goals and Objectives

Need	Objective	Evaluative measures
Project Goal 1a:		
Project Goal 1b:		
Project Goal 1c:		

Formative Evaluation Activities, Data, and Timeline

Program activity	Type of data and method of collection	Timeline

Forms

Excel Budget Template

		D	F	H	J	L
	HSI-STEM Budget	Year 1	Year 2	Year 3	Year 4	Year 5
		USDE	USDE	USDE	USDE	USDE
Fringe	**Personnel**					
	Project Administrators					
	Name					
	Project Director					
	Name					
0.38	Name/Rate of Pay/Effort					
	Title					
0.38	Name/Rate of Pay/Effort					
	Title					
0.095	Name/Rate of Pay/Effort					
	Title					
	Name/Rate of Pay/Effort					

(continued)

Forms

Excel Budget Template *(page 2 of 2)*

HSI-STEM Budget		D Year 1	F Year 2	H Year 3	J Year 4	L Year 5
Other than personnel services						
Travel						
	PD to Required Meeting					
	Professional Staff to Required Meetings					
Supplies and Materials						
	Lab/Research/Admin/Student Materials for SC					
Computers for Staff						
Software						
iPad Minis for Students						
Contractual	External Evaluators					
Total OTPS						
Total Direct						
Indirect @ ?%						
Student Stipends						
Total Project Costs						
Total Amount						

Glossary

Allocation: The amount of funds provided for a particular grant competition by the approving legislation and/or the amount of funds provided to a particular grantee.

Allowable costs: Budget expenses that are permitted by the legislation associated with the RFP. A list is usually detailed in the application materials.

Amendment: A change or addition to the proposal document initially submitted for funding. It can relate to a change in use of funds or office locations, activities, percent salary paid, number of employees or any other change. The request for permission to change would be sent to the program liaison.

Annual report: A yearly report submitted to funding agencies by the grantee following guidelines established by the grantor. Due dates and content of the report are specified by the grantor.

Application: The electronic document submitted by the institution/organization by the stated deadline containing all of the required assurances, forms, project narrative, budgets, and signatures required for the proposal to be considered.

Application notice: The official announcement of the grant competition published in the *Federal Register,* on the funder's website, and on Grants.gov or another website.

Application packet: The full details, including directions, assurances, forms, and budget documents that must be submitted in order to be considered for funding.

Assurances: The set of required forms, signed by the Authorized Institutional Representative, that pertain to institutional compliance with regulations associated with funding.

Authorization: The legislation enacted that authorizes the grant competition, includes the funds allocated for the overall competition, and stipulates the maximum allowable funding per award.

Authorized Institutional Representative (AIR): The person or persons at your institution/organization empowered to sign and submit proposals to funding agencies; also called the Authorized Signatory.

Boilerplate: Information describing your institution and its demographics that can be presented in several proposals. Using up-to-date information saves time and provides accurate and consistent information. Using an old proposal that is adapted for resubmission for a new competition almost always results in rejection.

Budget: The detailed presentation of how the funds will be spent in order to fulfill the components of the proposal. Contains information on personnel (including fringe benefits, salary rates, percent time worked) and on other than personnel services including books and materials to be purchased, equipment (if allowed), travel, computers, software, consulting services and indirect costs (institutional/organizational rate or mandated rate), stipends (if permitted), and total costs.

Budget narrative: A detailed explanation of each of the cost items in the budget with information on the roles and responsibilities of personnel and the need/reasons for other than personnel items.

Budget period: Usually a fiscal year. Most government grants use the federal fiscal year, October 1 to September 30.

Catalog of Federal Domestic Assistance (CFDA): A governmentwide compendium of federal programs, projects, and activities that provide assistance to the public. Each program has a unique CFDA identifier that can be used to search for information about the program (e.g., the identifier for Student Support Services is CFDA 84.042).

Code of Federal Regulations (CFR): The annual regulations and permanent rules that govern executive departments and agencies of the federal government and are published in the *Federal Register*.

Competitive priorities: These are supplemental priorities formulated by the USDE (available at **www.federalregister.gov/documents/2018/03/02/2018-04291/secretarys-final-supplemental-priorities-and-definitions-for-discretionary-grant-programs**) for which points are added to your basic score.

Conflict of interest: A conflict of interest occurs when an individual overseeing a grant (principal investigator, or PI) is in a position to personally benefit from decisions made with respect to the project.

Congressional district: Your institution/organization and/or the target population are located in a federal congressional district, which can be located at **https://house.gov/representatives/find**.

Continuation award: Most funding agencies award grants for multiple years (e.g,. 2016–2021, 2018–2022) but allocate the funding for 1 year at a time (see **Budget**

Period and **Project Period**). Each year of the project period the budget for that year is allocated.

Cost sharing: In order to assure the commitment of the grantee some agencies/RFPs ask that the institution/organization show the dollar amount they are allocating to the operation of the project. Actual funds or in-kind contributions are acceptable, but the RFP should be read carefully to determine what is mandated.

Deadline: The date and time that your proposal absolutely must be submitted according to the application guidelines. The relevant time stamp is not when you start the upload but when it is completed. For applications that are submitted online, the date and time stamp is applied when your application is fully uploaded. If there are many individuals trying to upload their applications at the same time, the system may be slow and the time stamp on your completed upload may be after the deadline. If this is the case, your application will not be eligible for review.

Direct cost: Those budget items that are related to personnel costs and other than personnel services costs. They are the costs of conducting the activities of the project.

Discretionary grant: Funds awarded on the basis of a competitive process in which a government agency reviews applications, using a formal review process based on legislative and regulatory requirements and published selection criteria.

Dissemination: The process of sharing the findings from your project with others through publications, presentations, workshops, and websites.

DUNS (Data Universal Numbering System) Number: This is a unique identifier for your institution/organization/company provided free by Dun and Bradstreet. It is required on applications and is used to predict financial stability and reliability.

Education Department General Administrative Regulations (EDGAR): Provide criteria and instruction on grant applications organized by grant categories.

Eligibility: Each discretionary grant competition RFP contains a section on types of institutions/organization entitled to apply. For example, Title V is a Strengthening Institutions Grant for Hispanic Serving Institutions (colleges and universities with 25% or more Hispanic enrollment).

Endowment: Some funders allow a percentage of the grant funds to be allocated to an established institutional/organizational endowment. These funds must be matched in full by new funds solicited from donors before they can be claimed, and only the accrued interest from the endowment can be expended.

Entity Identification Number (EIN): Also known as the Federal Employer Identification Number (FEIN) or the Federal Tax Identification Number, this is a unique nine-digit number assigned by the Internal Revenue Service to business entities in the United States for identification purposes.

Equipment: An item having a cost of more than $5,000 and a useful life of more than 1 year.

Evaluation: The process of determining whether activities/processes are carried out as specified in the proposal and whether the predicted outcomes are achieved.

Facilities and administrative costs: Also called indirect costs, these costs are for resources used mutually by different individuals and groups, making it difficult to assess precisely which users should pay what share. Institutions/organizations usually have a negotiated rate. Some discretionary grant competitions specify a cap on facilities and administrative costs.

Federal Register: The official journal of the federal government of the United States that contains government agency rules, proposed rules, and public notices. It is published daily, except on federal holidays, and can be accessed at **www.federal-register.gov**.

Final report: Funding agencies generally require that the grantee submit a final report at the end of the grant period that follows guidelines established by the grantor. Due dates and content of the report are specified by the grantor.

First-generation college student: Several discretionary grant competitions (e.g., all of the TRIO grants) specify that the project must serve low-income, first-generation students. Usually the RFP will define what is considered first generation. Typically, the TRIO programs require that neither parent has a baccalaureate degree in order to meet this priority. This is a subsection under Need for all of the TRIO RFPs, so the needs section of the proposal should include a chart or table, under the appropriate heading, that shows the levels of education of families in your service area.

Fiscal agent: The institution/organization responsible for the oversight of financial aspects of the grant budget. Assures that funds are spent according to the rules and regulations specified in the RFP.

Forecast of funding opportunities: A document that lists virtually all programs and competitions under which the Department of Education has invited or expects to invite applications for new awards and provides actual or estimated deadlines. Published yearly and accessible at **www2.ed.gov/fund/contract/find/forecast.html**.

Formative evaluation: Assessment that aims to determine if the implementation of the project is proceeding as described in the proposal and if modifications in the operation/activities are needed to achieve desired outcomes.

Fringe benefits: The other than salary costs associated with paying personnel working on the grant. Rates are usually set by the institution and can be provided by the Office of Grants and Contracts.

Grant: The funds awarded in response to a successful proposal; includes the regulations that govern the conduct of the project.

Grant Award Notification (GANS): This notice contains the funds awarded and the regulations pertaining to the award.

Grantee: The institution/organization receiving the funds.

Grantor: The agency, foundation, or corporation awarding the funds.

Grants officer: Also called the program/project liaison or officer. This is the individual at the funder who oversees your program and who can provide advice, approvals and information.

Grants.gov: One-stop website for finding funding opportunities and for developing and submitting an application for funding. In most institutions/organizations the authorized institutional representative must submit the final application.

Grants.gov tracking number: Once your application is submitted, a unique tracking number is assigned.

Guidelines: The RFP or Request for Proposal that specifies the application process and the proposal contents and regulations.

Indirect cost: Also referred to as overhead or administrative costs. It is the rate approved for your institution/organization, which specifies what budget costs are included in this category. Alternatively, indirect rates can be legislated as part of the RFP and capped at a percentage below that permitted to your institution. The legislated rate takes precedence.

Institutional review board (IRB): The IRB is the research ethics review board established by institutions/organizations to review projects that involve human subjects and determine if rules and regulations are followed.

Invitational priorities: These are supplemental priorities formulated by the USDE (available at **www.federalregister.gov/documents/2018/03/02/2018-04291/secretarys-final-supplemental-priorities-and-definitions-for-discretionary-grant-programs**) that dictate the focus of the proposal you submit.

Key personnel: These are individuals who contribute to the scientific development or execution of a project in a substantive, measurable way, including the principal investigator, project director/coordinator, instructor, and administrator.

Letter of inquiry: A letter of inquiry is sent to a foundation/corporation which does not review unsolicited proposals in order to present your ideas to them in the hope that they will see the value in them and invite your organization to submit a brief proposal. Note that some foundations/corporations clearly indicate that they do not accept letters of inquiry. The letter of inquiry should be considered a marketing document intended to pique the interest of those who review it. The first section of the letter should contain information about your organization and your funding purpose. The second section should explicitly connect your purpose to the purpose of the foundation. A final section should provide estimated funding that is within the amount provided by the foundation/corporation for projects funded in the past (information that is usually available on their website).

Letter of intent: Can be required or optional. When optional, it enables funders to determine about how many applications to expect and in what areas. When required, it is used for a similar purpose, but an entity cannot submit a proposal unless it has completed an LOI. Also, some funders use the LOI to determine who they will invite to apply for the competition based on whether the purpose reviewed in the LOI matches the funder's areas of interest.

Letter of support: This is sometimes required so that funders can determine whether the support and/or partnerships and collaborations detailed in the proposal are genuine. Letters should detail what the writer will bring to the project in time, money, facilities, and participation.

Logic model: A framework used by funders, managers, and evaluators of programs to evaluate the effectiveness of a program. It can also be used during planning and implementation of a program. See, for example, **http://toolkit.pellinstitute.org/evaluation-guide/plan-budget/using-a-logic-model**.

Low-income: Several discretionary grant competitions (e.g., all of the TRIO grants) specify that the project must serve low-income, first-generation students. Usually the RFP will define what is considered low-income. Typically the TRIO programs use 150% of the poverty level and publish the income level that meets this priority. This is a subsection under "Need" for all of the TRIO RFPs, so the needs section of the proposal should include a chart or table under the appropriate heading that shows how many individuals/families in your service area meet this requirement.

Memorandum of understanding (MOU): Partners or collaborators in your proposal should sign a prepared document that details their roles and responsibilities in the project.

Need statement: The section of the proposal in which you provide evidence that the area and participants you will serve meet the need requirements detailed in the RFP. This could be low-income, ethnicity, first-generation college students, or other need requirements.

Outcomes: The resulting achievements of your project as specified by your objectives and evaluation measures.

Overhead/indirect/administrative costs: Also referred to as indirect costs or facilities and administrative costs, they are based on the direct costs of the project and determined by the approved rate for the institution/organization or a maximum rate dictated by the RFP or funder.

Participant(s): The individual or individuals being served by your project. In many cases they must meet RFP requirements for participation.

Participant support costs: These are direct costs for items such as stipends or subsistence allowances, travel allowances, and registration fees paid to or on behalf of participants or trainees (but not employees) in connection with conferences or training projects.

Peer reviewer: An individual who reviews and scores submitted proposals using a scoring rubric.

Principal investigator (PI): The individual who is responsible for oversight of the grant and accountable for financial and program aspects of the project.

Prior approval: Any substantive changes made to a project after it is funded must be approved by the funder's program officer or project liaison.

Process evaluation: An assessment that aims to determine if the implementation of the project is proceeding as described in the proposal and if modifications in the operation/activities are needed to achieve desired outcomes.

Product evaluation: The achievement of your project objectives as measured by the outcome measures, usually reported annually and summarized at the end of the project period.

Program officer/liaison: The person or persons at the funding agency who respond to your inquiries and oversee your project, approving requested modifications, making site visits, reviewing your annual fiscal and program reports, monitoring the progress of your project, and assigning prior experience points (for TRIO grants) when you apply for the next competition.

Program/project: The activities, evaluations, and other aspects you will implement during you conduct of the approved proposal.

Project director: The person who is likely in charge of the day-to-day operations of the project; reports to the principal investigator and oversees the work of the individuals who implement the activities.

Project narrative: The proposal submitted to the funding agency as part of the application package. Follows the outline provided by the selection criteria and adheres to all the formatting regulations included in the RFP.

Project period: The number of years of project support anticipated if all requirements continue to be met by the institution/organization (e.g., TRIO grants are awarded for a 5-year project period with yearly budget allocations).

Proposal: The narrative section of the application, organized according to the selection criteria and adhering to all required formatting instructions.

Qualitative measurement: Qualitative data encompasses text, words, and data defined as nominal or ordinal scale data. Must be analyzed using nonparametric tests.

Quantitative measurement: Qualitative data has numerical values and uses an interval or ratio scale. Can be analyzed using parametric statistical tests.

Request for Application (RFA): A Request for Application is issued by funders who have an allocation earmarked for particular types of programs/services.

Request for Proposal (RFP): A Request for Proposal is issued by funders who have an allocation earmarked for particular types of programs/services.

Review/selection criteria: The published listing of specific information that funders are requesting be included in the proposal. The selection criteria should be used as the table of contents and the section headings in the proposal.

Senate district: The district in which your institution/organization and/or the target population is located. You can determine your senate district at **www.senate.gov/senators/contact.**

Single–state point of contact: In some states notification that your institution has submitted an application to the federal government in response to an RFP must be submitted to the Single State Point of Contact. Your Office of Research and Sponsored Programs will know if this is the case for your state, or you can find a listing on the Internet.

Site Visit: Your project liaison or other representative from the funding agency may schedule a visit to your program to assess your adherence to the proposal that was approved in order to assist you in improving the program or to determine if your program is proceeding on track. After the visit, a letter detailing the findings will be sent, and you may have to respond to show how you have resolved any issues that were noted during the visit.

Stipend: A sum paid to a program participant based on meeting certain program participation requirements. Stipends are not included in the total direct costs used to calculate the indirect costs.

Subcontract: For a project that involves more than one institution/organization or employs consultants or external evaluators, a subcontract may be executed and the funds for the consultant(s) or evaluator(s) are set aside in the budget documents or transferred to the subcontractor. Most times an independent contractor agreement must be completed to assure that the individuals cannot be classified as employees.

Summative evaluation: The yearly outcomes of the project entail determination of the extent to which the proposed objectives have been met according to the measures proposed (also applicable to the final project outcomes determined at the end of the project period).

Supplies: Purchased items under the Other Than Personnel Services budget section that have a life of less than 1 year, are consumable, and cost under $5,000.

Sustainability: The extent to which the activities and support of your project will be continued after the project period concludes. Will personnel costs be borne by the institution/organization? Will support systems for students be continued? Will innovative instructional methods continue to be implemented? Will the methods and activities of your project be implemented by others in your organization?

Table of contents: The table of contents for your proposal should be organized by the selection criteria presented in the RFP. Tables, charts, and figures should be added under the specific section in which they are contained.

Target group: Individuals with specific characteristics who will be served by the project. Sometimes these are dictated by the RFP (e.g., TRIO grants serve low-income, first-generation college students) HSI: STEM grants serve students at Hispanic-serving institutions preparing for majors/careers in science, technology, engineering, or mathematics.

Technical assistance: Funding agencies are required by statute to offer technical assistance to institutions/organizations who are planning to prepare applications to their competitions, in the form of workshops, and most recently online webinars. Some educational organizations will offer proposal-writing workshops to members to help them prepare competitive proposals. Some of these are funded by training grants provided by funding agencies. For example, the Council for Opportunity in Education (**www.coenet.us**) offers proposal-writing workshops in the years that TRIO grants are due.

Terms of award: When the funding notification is received or posted online, it contains the terms under which the award is provided. This includes the legal requirements imposed on a federal government grant by statute, regulation, policy, or other source of authority referenced in the Notice of Award.

Timeline: The comprehensive and detailed schedule of when activities for your project will take place. The more detailed the timeline, the better sense the peer reviewer has that you have thought through issues and deadlines pertaining to the implementation of the project.

Total direct costs: The total costs of project implementation prior to adding on the indirect costs.

Unallowable costs: Budget expenses that are *not* permitted by the legislation associated with the RFP. A list is usually provided in the application materials.

Underserved population: A group of individuals who have limited access to opportunities and services.

USDE: United States Department of Education (**www.ed.gov**).

Using Action Verbs to Engage the Reader

Henriette Anne Klauser, in *Writing on Both Sides of the Brain* (1986), has commented on the use of passive voice:

> The passive voice is convoluted; it takes the energy out of your writing and makes your message flaccid. It is absolutely homicidal—it kills the people in your prose. . . . The passive voice invariably comes across as pontificating, patronizing, talking down. It sounds insincere, even dishonest, and it makes the reader uncomfortable, not trusting, though usually the reader cannot put her finger on why.

Action verbs also serve to promote concise and persuasive grant proposals and help the external reader to engage with your project.

For this reason the grant writer should always use an active voice and picture words and action verbs.

Achieve	Belong	Elevate
Allow	Bring	Engage
Analyze	Change	Ensure
Announce	Choose	Entail
Appeal	Clarify	Envision
Apply	Coach	Equal
Assess	Combine	Establish
Assist	Compare	Evaluate
Balance	Direct	Excel
Become	Discuss	Exemplify
Begin	Distinguish	Exhibit
Believe	Educate	Experiment

Explain	Move	Reveal
Extend	Negotiate	Review
Find	Need	Sample
Focus	Observe	Search
Form	Occur	Send
Investigate	Offer	Show
Involve	Operate	Signal
Know	Organize	Specify
Lack	Perform	Start
Lead	Plan	State
Learn	Report	Suggest
Maintain	Research	Support
Make	Restore	Survey
Manage	Result	Synthesize
Modify	Return	Taught
Motivate	Require	

For those of you who wish to explore other active verbs that can be used to enliven your grant proposals, a search for "action verbs for grant writing" on Google or other search engines will provide more examples.

APPENDIX B

Web Resources

General

Grant Writing 101—USDE
www2.ed.gov/about/offices/list/osdfs/grantwrite101.pdf

Purdue Online Writing Lab
http://owl.english.purdue.edu

Grant Writing: How to Write and Search for Grants
https://nonprofitquarterly.org/2017/04/01/grant-writing-how-to-write-grant-proposal/

How to Write a Grant Proposal
www.arc.gov/funding/HowtoWriteaGrantProposal.asp

How to Write a Winning Grant Proposal in 11 Steps
www.thebalance.com/how-to-write-a-grant-proposal-2501980

Proposal Resources
www.chaffey.edu/grants/common.shtml#narrative

Online Course for Proposal Writing
https://grantspace.org/training/topics/proposal-writing

Tips for Project Planning and Proposal Writing
www2.sfasu.edu/orsp/tam_part3.html#tips
Social Science Research Council

The Art of Writing Proposals
https://guides.lib.umich.edu/c.php?g=283181&p=1886514
University of Michigan

The Proposal Writer's Guide
**https://orsp.umich.edu/sites/default/files/resource-download/
proposal-writers-guide-final.pdf**

Chapters 1 and 2

Proposal Writing Flow Chart
www.pacificu.edu/search/site/proposal%20%20process

Proposal Writing: Stages and Strategies with Examples
www.studygs.net/proposal.htm

Chapter 3

How to Write Successful Collaborative Applications
**https://granttrainingcenter.com/blog/write-successful-collaborative-
application**

Collaborative Proposal Development Resources
**www.washington.edu/research/collaboration/collaborative-proposal-
resources**

Chapter 4

A Winning Strategy for Grant Applications: Focus on Impact
**www.the-scientist.com/profession/a-winning-strategy-for-grant-
applications-focus-on-impact-57515**

Checklist for Grant Writers

**www.imls.gov/sites/default/files/legacy/assets/1/AssetManager/
AAHC_Convening_Toolkit2.pdf**

Consensus Building

http://web.mit.edu/publicdisputes/practice/cbh_ch1.html

**www.leadstrat.com/blog/the-art-of-getting-to-yes-5-techniques-
for-building-consensus-2**

Multi-Attribute Consensus Building Tool

https://nceo.umn.edu/docs/Tools/MACBtool.pdf

Build Consensus

www.skymark.com/resources/tools/building_consensus.asp

Core Facilitation Tools

https://seedsforchange.org.uk/tools.pdf

Facilitator Tool Kit

**https://oqi.wisc.edu/resourcelibrary/uploads/resources/
Facilitator%20Tool%20Kit.pdf**

Chapter 5

Approaching Foundations

**https://grantspace.org/resources/knowledge-base/approaching-
foundations**

Finding Funding for your Research

www.g5.gov
www.grants.gov/applicants/apply-for-grants.html
**https://oedb.org/ilibrarian/100_places_to_find_funding_your_
research**

Chapter 7

Common Components of Grant Proposals

**www.usi.edu/ospra/grant-proposal-and-federal-contract-
development/common-components-of-grant-proposals**

Components of a Grant Proposal

**https://valenciacollege.edu/academic-affairs/resource-development/
documents/proposal-components_71812_000.pdf**

Writing a Grant Proposal

www.communitygrantsnow.com/2011/02/07/writing-the-narrative

Common Elements in a Grant Proposal—Chaffey College

www.chaffey.edu/grants/common.shtml

Chapter 8

Writing a Compelling Grant Abstract

**https://your.yale.edu/sites/default/files/files/
HowToWriteACompellingAbstractForGrantApplication_July2017.pdf**

Elements of a Good Proposal Abstract

**http://grant-central-station.com/articles/the-elements-of-a-good-
proposal-abstract**

Creating a Grant Abstract

**https://your.yale.edu/sites/default/files/
HowToWriteACompellingAbstractForGrantApplication_July2017.pdf**

Chapter 9

W. K. Kellogg Foundation Logic Model Manual

www.wkkf.org/-/media/pdfs/logicmodel.pdf

University of Wisconsin-Extension—Logic Model

https://fyi.uwex.edu/programdevelopment/logic-models

University of Wisconsin-Extension—Logic Model Course

https://fyi.uwex.edu/programdevelopment/logic-models
**https://fyi.uwex.edu/programdevelopment/files/2016/03/
lmcourseall.pdf**
**https://fyi.uwex.edu/programdevelopment/files/2016/03/
lmguidecomplete.pdf**
**https://fyi.uwex.edu/programdevelopment/files/2016/03/LM_
WorksheetCSREESTableformat.doc**

Logic Models: A Tool for Effective Program Planning, Collaboration, and Monitoring

http://files.eric.ed.gov/fulltext/ED544779.pdf

Pell Institute Logic Model

http://toolkit.pellinstitute.org/evaluation-guide/plan-budget/using-a-logic-model

Chapter 10

How to Write a Needs Statement

www.thebalance.com/how-to-write-a-need-statement-for-your-grant-proposal-2501959

The Need Statement

www.dhs.state.il.us/page.aspx?item=4803

Writing the Needs or Problem Statement

www.sagepub.com/sites/default/files/upm-binaries/15910_Chapter_5.pdf

Chapter 11

Writing Goals and Objectives

www.niu.edu/facdev/_pdf/guide/prepare/writing_goals_and_objectives.pdf

How to Write Goals and Objectives for Grant Proposals

www.bpcc.edu/grantsexternalfunding/goalsobjectives.html

Writing Measurable Goals and Objectives

www.asha.org/uploadedFiles/Writing-Measurable-Goals-and-Objectives.pdf

How to Write SMART Goals

www.smartsheet.com/blog/essential-guide-writing-smart-goals

Writing Goals for Grant Proposals

www.thebalance.com/writing-goals-for-grant-proposal-2501951

How to Write SMART Goals and Objectives
www.cognology.com.au/learning_center/howtowritesmartobj

Chapter 12

Institute for Student Achievement
www.studentachievement.org

Developing a Program Assessment Plan
www.cmich.edu/search/Pages/default.aspx?k=developing%20a%20 program%20assessment%20plan

Software for Creating Figures and Charts
www.smartdraw.com
www.organimi.com
www.lucidchart.com
www.orgplus.com

How to Compose Your Grant Application's Management Plan
www.brown.edu/research/conducting-research-brown/preparing-proposal/proposal-development-services/writing-management-plan

How to Write the Personnel Narrative on Your Grant Application
https://osp.mit.edu/grant-and-contract-administration/managing-projects/key-personnel

Chapter 13

Institute of Education Sciences
https://ies.ed.gov

Institute of Education Sciences: What Works Clearinghouse
https://ies.ed.gov/ncee/wwc

The Step-by-Step Guide to Evaluation
http://ww2.wkkf.org/digital/evaluationguide/main.html

Pell Institute Evaluation Toolkit

**http://toolkit.pellinstitute.org/evaluation-guide/plan-budget/
choose-an-evaluation-design**

Tools for Grantees: Evaluation

**https://wp.stolaf.edu/ir-e/resources-for-faculty-and-staff/grant-
project-evaluation**

**https://ed.sc.gov/finance/grants/scde-grants-program-planning-
tools-templates-and-samples/grant-program-evaluation**

Chapter 14

Allowable and Unallowable Expenditures

**www.mtholyoke.edu/sites/default/files/sponsoredresearch/docs/
Allowable_Unallowable_Expenditures_on_Federal_Grants.pdf**

Developing a Proposal Budget

www.rit.edu/research/srs/proposalprep/howto_budget

Writing a Budget Narrative/Justification

www.rit.edu/research/srs/proposalprep/budget_narrative

The Who, What, When, Where, and How of Grant Budgets

www.grantadviser.com/budget

Introduction to Project Budgets

https://grantspace.org/training/introduction-to-project-budgets

Chapter 15

Research Dissemination

https://guides.library.vcu.edu/dissemination/template

Grant Writing: Focus on the Lasting Impact of the Funder's Investment

**www.fasttrackimpact.com/single-post/2016/02/14/Pathways-
to-topscoring-impacts-an-analysis-of-%E2%80%98pathways-to-
impact%E2%80%99-in-grant-applications-that-led-to-highly-
scored-impact-case-studies**

Program Sustainability Assessment Tool

https://sustaintool.org/understand

How to Write the Sustainability Section of a Proposal

www.tools4dev.org/resources/how-to-write-the-sustainability-section-of-a-proposal

Beyond the Grant: Planning for Sustainability

https://grantproseinc.com/wp-content/uploads/2013/07/GrantProse_Planning_for_Sustainability.pdf

General Sustainability

extension.missouri.edu/4hlife/documents/sustain/GeneralSustainabilityPresentation.ppt

Two Tips on How to Write the Significance of the Study

https://simplyeducate.me/2015/02/09/two-tips-on-how-to-write-the-significance-of-the-study

Significance of the Problem

www.rachellocke.com/s/Significance_steps-to-write_R_Locke_v102317.pdf

NIH Grant Writing Tips: The Significance of "Significance"

https://morganonscience.com/grantwriting/nih-grant-writing-tips-the-significance-of-significance

Chapter 16

What Is the Point of an "Invitational Priority?"

www.newamerica.org/education-policy/early-elementary-education-policy/early-ed-watch/what-is-the-point-of-an-invitational-priority

U.S. ED Releases Proposed Priorities for Competitive Grant Programs

https://education.ufl.edu/educational-research/10775

Final USDE Priorities for Competitive Grant Programs

https://blog.ed.gov/2017/10/ed-releases-secretarys-proposed-priorities-competitive-grant-programs

www.federalregister.gov/documents/2017/10/12/2017-22127/secretarys-proposed-supplemental-priorities-and-definitions-for-discretionary-grant-programs

Use of Evidence in 5 Largest Competitive Grant Programs

www.fundingcentre.com.au/help/using-evidence

Characteristics of Studies that Might Meet WWC Standards

www2.ed.gov/programs/triotalent/wwc-standards.ppt

Talent Search Studies for Competitive Preference Priorities

www2.ed.gov/programs/triotalent/ts-studies-for-cpps.doc

Chapter 17

OPE Peer Reviewers: Frequently Asked Questions

www2.ed.gov/about/offices/list/ope/peer-reviewers/faq.html

Become a Grant Reviewer

www.xavier.edu/grant-services/documents/BecomeaGrantReviewer.pdf

Chapter 18

Grant Tips

www.hrsa.gov/sites/default/files/grants/apply/writestrong/grantwritingtips.pdf

Do's and Don'ts of Grant Writing

http://nonprofitinformation.com/grant-writing-tip

Grant Writing Tips

www.southernsare.org/Grants/Writing-Your-Grant

Grant Writing Tips

www.acf.hhs.gov/fysb/resource/grant-writing-tips

10 Tips for Successful Grant Writing
www.chronicle.com/article/10-Tips-for-Successful-Grant/242535

Science magazine series: How Not to Kill a Grant Application

Part 1 Murder Most Foul: **www.sciencemag.org/careers/2000/01/murder-most-foul-how-not-kill-grant-application**

Part 2 Abstract Killers: **www.sciencemag.org/careers/2000/01/abstract-killers-how-not-kill-grant-application-part-two**

Part 3 So What?: **www.sciencemag.org/careers/2000/02/so-what-how-not-kill-grant-application-part-three**

Part 4 Lost at Sea: **www.sciencemag.org/careers/2000/02/lost-sea-how-not-kill-grant-application-part-four**

Part 5 The Facts of the Case Thusfar: **www.sciencemag.org/careers/2000/05/how-not-kill-grant-application-part-five-facts-case-thus-far**

Part 6 Developing Your Research Plan: **www.sciencemag.org/careers/2000/08/how-not-kill-grant-application-part-6-developing-your-research-plan**

APPENDIX C

Examples of Selection Criteria

This appendix includes examples of the selection criteria, including point values, for three TRIO competitions: Talent Search, Student Support Services, and HSI-STEM. These can be found in the *Federal Register* announcements and/or in the application materials posted on the specific USDE websites for the particular RFPs.

As noted previously, I find it very helpful to create a word-processing document using these selection criteria as the section headings for both the table of contents and the project narrative. As you can see from Figure 17.1, these criteria are exactly what the reader uses to score your proposal. If your project narrative is in the same order as the scoring material, the reader does not have to search for your responses—they are right in the same order as his or her worksheet.

As readers have to complete thoughtful reviews on several proposals in a short period of time, anything the writer can do to assist their work will be greatly appreciated.

Appendix C1: Talent Search

§ 643.21 What selection criteria does the Secretary use?

The Secretary uses the following criteria to evaluate an application for a new grant:

(a) *Need for the project* (24 points). The Secretary evaluates the need for a Talent Search project in the proposed target area on the basis of the extent to which the application contains clear evidence of the following:

  (1) (4 points) A high number or high percentage of the following—

    (i) Low-income families residing in the target area; or

(ii) Students attending the target schools who are eligible for free or reduced priced lunch as described in sections 9(b)(1) and 17(c)(4) of the Richard B. Russell National School Lunch Act.

(2) (2 points) Low rates of high school persistence among individuals in the target schools as evidenced by the annual student persistence rates in the proposed target schools for the most recent year for which data are available.

(3) (4 points) Low rates of students in the target school or schools who graduate high school with a regular secondary school diploma in the standard number of years for the most recent year for which data are available.

(4) (6 points) Low postsecondary enrollment and completion rates among individuals in the target area and schools as evidenced by—

(i) Low rates of enrollment in programs of postsecondary education by graduates of the target schools in the most recent year for which data are available; and

(ii) A high number or high percentage of individuals residing in the target area with education completion levels below the baccalaureate degree level.

(5) (2 points) The extent to which the target secondary schools do not offer their students the courses or academic support to complete a rigorous secondary school program of study or have low participation or low success by low-income or first generation students in such courses.

(6) (6 points) Other indicators of need for a TS project, including low academic achievement and low standardized test scores of students enrolled in the target schools, a high ratio of students to school counselors in the target schools, and the presence of unaddressed academic or socio-economic problems of eligible individuals, including foster care youth and homeless children and youth in the target schools or the target area.

(b) *Objectives* (8 points). The Secretary evaluates the quality of the applicant's objectives and proposed targets (percentages) in the following areas on the basis of the extent to which they are both ambitious, as related to the need data provided under paragraph (a) of this section, and attainable, given the project's plan of operation, budget, and other resources:

(1) (2 points) Secondary school persistence.

(2) (2 points) Secondary school graduation (regular secondary school diploma).

(3) (1 point) Secondary school graduation (rigorous secondary school program of study).

(4) (2 points) Postsecondary education enrollment.

(5) (1 point) Postsecondary degree attainment.

(c) *Plan of operation* (30 points). The Secretary evaluates the quality of the applicant's plan of operation on the basis of the following:

(1) (3 points) The plan to inform the residents, schools, and community organizations in the target area of the purpose, objectives, and services of the project and the eligibility requirements for participation in the project.

(2) (3 points) The plan to identify and select eligible project participants.

(3) (10 points) The plan for providing the services delineated in § 643.4 as appropriate based on the project's assessment of each participant's need for services.

(4) (6 points) The plan to work in a coordinated, collaborative, and cost-effective manner as part of an overarching college access strategy with the target schools or school system and other programs for disadvantaged students to provide participants with access to and assistance in completing a rigorous secondary school program of study.

(5) (6 points) The plan, including timelines, personnel, and other resources, to ensure the proper and efficient administration of the project, including the project's organizational structure; the time commitment of key project staff; and financial, personnel, and records management.

(6) (2 points) The plan to follow former participants as they enter, continue in, and complete postsecondary education.

(d) *Applicant and community support* (16 points). The Secretary evaluates the applicant and community support for the proposed project on the basis of the extent to which the applicant has made provision for resources to supplement the grant and enhance the project's services, including—

(1) (8 points) Facilities, equipment, supplies, personnel, and other resources committed by the applicant; and

(2) (8 points) Resources secured through written commitments from community partners.

(i) An applicant that is an institution of higher education must include in its application commitments from the target schools and community organizations;

(ii) An applicant that is a secondary school must include in its commitments from institutions of higher education, community organizations, and, as appropriate, other secondary schools and the school district; and

(iii) An applicant that is a community organization must include in its application commitments from the target schools and institutions of higher education.

(e) *Quality of personnel* (9 points).

(1) The Secretary evaluates the quality of the personnel the applicant plans to use in the project on the basis of the following:

(i) The qualifications required of the project director.

(ii) The qualifications required of each of the other personnel to be used in the project.

(iii) The plan to employ personnel who have succeeded in overcoming the disadvantages of circumstances like those of the population of the target area.

(2) In evaluating the qualifications of a person, the Secretary considers his or her experience and training in fields related to the objectives of the project.

(f) *Budget* (5 points). The Secretary evaluates the extent to which the project budget is reasonable, cost-effective, and adequate to support the project.

(g) *Evaluation plan* (8 points). The Secretary evaluates the quality of the evaluation plan for the project on the basis of the extent to which the applicant's methods of evaluation—

(1) Are appropriate to the project's objectives;

(2) Provide for the applicant to determine, using specific and quantifiable measures, the success of the project in—

(i) Making progress toward achieving its objectives (a formative evaluation); and

(ii) Achieving its objectives at the end of the project period (a summative evaluation); and

(3) Provide for the disclosure of unanticipated project outcomes, using quantifiable measures if appropriate.

Appendix C2: Student Support Services

§ 646.21 What selection criteria does the Secretary use to evaluate an application?

The Secretary uses the following criteria to evaluate an application for a new grant:

(a) *Need for the project* (24 points). The Secretary evaluates the need for a Student Support Services project proposed at the applicant institution on the basis of the extent to which the application contains clear evidence of—

(1) (8 points) A high number or percentage, or both, of students enrolled or accepted for enrollment at the applicant institution who meet the eligibility requirements of § 646.3;

(2) (8 points) The academic and other problems that eligible students encounter at the applicant institution; and

(3) (8 points) The differences between eligible Student Support Services students compared to an appropriate group, based on the following indicators:

   (i) Retention and graduation rates.

   (ii) Grade point averages.

   (iii) Graduate and professional school enrollment rates (four-year colleges only).

   (iv) Transfer rates from two-year to four-year institutions (two-year colleges only).

(b) *Objectives* (8 points). The Secretary evaluates the quality of the applicant's proposed objectives in the following areas on the basis of the extent to which they are both ambitious, as related to the need data provided under paragraph (a) of this section, and attainable, given the project's plan of operation, budget, and other resources.

(1) (3 points) Retention in postsecondary education.

(2) (2 points) In good academic standing at grantee institution.

(3) Two-year institutions only.

   (i) (1 point) Certificate or degree completion; and

   (ii) (2 points) Certificate or degree completion and transfer to a four-year institution.

(4) Four-year institutions only. (3 points) Completion of a baccalaureate degree.

(c) *Plan of operation* (30 points). The Secretary evaluates the quality of the applicant's plan of operation on the basis of the following:

(1) (3 points) The plan to inform the institutional community (students, faculty, and staff) of the goals, objectives, and services of the project and the eligibility requirements for participation in the project.

(2) (3 points) The plan to identify, select, and retain project participants with academic need.

(3) (4 points) The plan for assessing each individual participant's need for specific services and monitoring his or her academic progress at the institution to ensure satisfactory academic progress.

(4) (10 points) The plan to provide services that address the goals and objectives of the project.

(5) (10 points) The applicant's plan to ensure proper and efficient administration of the project, including the organizational placement of the project; the time commitment of key project staff; the specific plans for financial management, student records management, and personnel management; and, where appropriate, its plan for coordination with other programs for disadvantaged students.

(d) *Institutional commitment* (16 points). The Secretary evaluates the institutional commitment to the proposed project on the basis of the extent to which the applicant has—

(1) (6 points) Committed facilities, equipment, supplies, personnel, and other resources to supplement the grant and enhance project services;

(2) (6 points) Established administrative and academic policies that enhance participants' retention at the institution and improve their chances of graduating from the institution;

(3) (2 points) Demonstrated a commitment to minimize the dependence on student loans in developing financial aid packages for project participants by committing institutional resources to the extent possible; and

(4) (2 points) Assured the full cooperation and support of the Admissions, Student Aid, Registrar and data collection and analysis components of the institution.

(e) *Quality of personnel* (9 points). To determine the quality of personnel the applicant plans to use, the Secretary looks for information that shows—

(1) (3 points) The qualifications required of the project director, including formal education and training in fields related to the objectives of the project, and experience in designing, managing, or implementing Student Support Services or similar projects;

(2) (3 points) The qualifications required of other personnel to be used in the project, including formal education, training, and work experience in fields related to the objectives of the project; and

(3) (3 points) The quality of the applicant's plan for employing personnel who have succeeded in overcoming barriers similar to those confronting the project's target population.

(f) *Budget* (5 points). The Secretary evaluates the extent to which the project budget is reasonable, cost-effective, and adequate to support the project.

(g) *Evaluation plan* (8 points). The Secretary evaluates the quality of the evaluation plan for the project on the basis of the extent to which—

(1) The applicant's methods for evaluation—

(i) (2 points) Are appropriate to the project and include both quantitative and qualitative evaluation measures; and

(ii) (2 points) Examine in specific and measurable ways, using appropriate baseline data, the success of the project in improving academic achievement, retention and graduation of project participants; and

(2) (4 points) The applicant intends to use the results of an evaluation to make programmatic changes based upon the results of project evaluation.

Appendix C3: HSI-STEM

§ 34 CFR 75.210 General selection criteria.

In determining the selection criteria to evaluate applications submitted in a grant competition, the Secretary may select one or more of the following criteria and may select from among the list of optional factors under each criterion. The Secretary may define a selection criterion by selecting one or more specific factors within a criterion or assigning factors from one criterion to another criterion.

(a) *Need for project.*

(1) The Secretary considers the need for the proposed project.

(2) In determining the need for the proposed project, the Secretary considers one or more of the following factors:

(i) The magnitude or severity of the problem to be addressed by the proposed project.

(ii) The magnitude of the need for the services to be provided or the activities to be carried out by the proposed project.

(iii) The extent to which the proposed project will provide services or otherwise address the needs of students at risk of educational failure.

(iv) The extent to which the proposed project will focus on serving or otherwise addressing the needs of disadvantaged individuals.

(v) The extent to which specific gaps or weaknesses in services, infrastructure, or opportunities have been identified and will be addressed by the proposed project, including the nature and magnitude of those gaps or weaknesses.

(vi) The extent to which the proposed project will prepare personnel for fields in which shortages have been demonstrated.

(b) *Significance.*

(1) The Secretary considers the significance of the proposed project.

(2) In determining the significance of the proposed project, the Secretary considers one or more of the following factors:

(i) The national significance of the proposed project.

(ii) The significance of the problem or issue to be addressed by the proposed project.

(iii) The potential contribution of the proposed project to increased knowledge or understanding of educational problems, issues, or effective strategies.

(iv) The potential contribution of the proposed project to increased knowledge or understanding of rehabilitation problems, issues, or effective strategies.

(v) The likelihood that the proposed project will result in system change or improvement.

(vi) The potential contribution of the proposed project to the development and advancement of theory, knowledge, and practices in the field of study.

(vii) The potential for generalizing from the findings or results of the proposed project.

(viii) The extent to which the proposed project is likely to yield findings that may be utilized by other appropriate agencies and organizations.

(ix) The extent to which the proposed project is likely to build local capacity to provide, improve, or expand services that address the needs of the target population.

(x) The extent to which the proposed project involves the development or demonstration of promising new strategies that build on, or are alternatives to, existing strategies.

(xi) The likely utility of the products (such as information, materials, processes, or techniques) that will result from the proposed project, including the potential for their being used effectively in a variety of other settings.

(xii) The extent to which the results of the proposed project are to be disseminated in ways that will enable others to use the information or strategies.

(xiii) The potential replicability of the proposed project or strategies, including, as appropriate, the potential for implementation in a variety of settings.

(xiv) The importance or magnitude of the results or outcomes likely to be attained by the proposed project, especially improvements in teaching and student achievement.

(xv) The importance or magnitude of the results or outcomes likely to be attained by the proposed project, especially improvements in employment, independent living services, or both, as appropriate.

(xvi) The importance or magnitude of the results or outcomes likely to be attained by the proposed project.

(c) *Quality of the project design.*

(1) The Secretary considers the quality of the design of the proposed project.

(2) In determining the quality of the design of the proposed project, the Secretary considers one or more of the following factors:

(i) The extent to which the goals, objectives, and outcomes to be achieved by the proposed project are clearly specified and measurable.

(ii) The extent to which the design of the proposed project is appropriate to, and will successfully address, the needs of the target population or other identified needs.

(iii) The extent to which there is a conceptual framework underlying the proposed research or demonstration activities and the quality of that framework.

(iv) The extent to which the proposed activities constitute a coherent, sustained program of research and development in the field, including, as appropriate, a substantial addition to an ongoing line of inquiry.

(v) The extent to which the proposed activities constitute a coherent, sustained program of training in the field.

(vi) The extent to which the proposed project is based upon a specific research design, and the quality and appropriateness of that design, including the scientific rigor of the studies involved.

(vii) The extent to which the proposed research design includes a thorough, high-quality review of the relevant literature, a high-quality plan for research activities, and the use of appropriate theoretical and methodological tools, including those of a variety of disciplines, if appropriate.

(viii) The extent to which the design of the proposed project includes a thorough, high-quality review of the relevant literature, a high-quality plan for project implementation, and the use of appropriate methodological tools to ensure successful achievement of project objectives.

(ix) The quality of the proposed demonstration design and procedures for documenting project activities and results.

(x) The extent to which the design for implementing and evaluating the proposed project will result in information to guide possible replication of project activities or strategies, including information about the effectiveness of the approach or strategies employed by the project.

(xi) The extent to which the proposed development efforts include adequate quality controls and, as appropriate, repeated testing of products.

(xii) The extent to which the proposed project is designed to build capacity and yield results that will extend beyond the period of Federal financial assistance.

(xiii) The extent to which the design of the proposed project reflects up-to-date knowledge from research and effective practice.

(xiv) The extent to which the proposed project represents an exceptional approach for meeting statutory purposes and requirements.

(xv) The extent to which the proposed project represents an exceptional approach to the priority or priorities established for the competition.

(xvi) The extent to which the proposed project will integrate with or build on similar or related efforts to improve relevant outcomes (as defined in 34 CFR 77.1(c)), using existing funding streams from other programs or policies supported by community, State, and Federal resources.

(xvii) The extent to which the proposed project will establish linkages with other appropriate agencies and organizations providing services to the target population.

(xviii) The extent to which the proposed project is part of a comprehensive effort to improve teaching and learning and support rigorous academic standards for students.

(xix) The extent to which the proposed project encourages parental involvement.

(xx) The extent to which the proposed project encourages consumer involvement.

(xxi) The extent to which performance feedback and continuous improvement are integral to the design of the proposed project.

(xxii) The quality of the methodology to be employed in the proposed project.

(xxiii) The extent to which fellowship recipients or other project participants are to be selected on the basis of academic excellence.

(xxiv) The extent to which the applicant demonstrates that it has the resources to operate the project beyond the length of the grant, including a multi-year financial and operating model and accompanying plan; the demonstrated commitment of any partners; evidence of broad support from stakeholders (e.g., State educational agencies, teachers' unions) critical to the project's long-term success; or more than one of these types of evidence.

(xxv) The potential and planning for the incorporation of project purposes, activities, or benefits into the ongoing work of the applicant beyond the end of the grant.

(xxvi) The extent to which the proposed project will increase efficiency in the use of time, staff, money, or other resources in order to improve results and increase productivity.

(xxvii) The extent to which the proposed project will integrate with or build on similar or related efforts in order to improve relevant outcomes (as defined in 34 CFR 77.1(c)), using nonpublic funds or resources.

(xxviii) The extent to which the proposed project is supported by evidence of promise (as defined in 34 CFR 77.1(c)).(xxix) The extent to which the proposed project is supported by strong theory (as defined in 34 CFR 77.1

(d) *Quality of project services.*

(1) The Secretary considers the quality of the services to be provided by the proposed project.

(2) In determining the quality of the services to be provided by the proposed project, the Secretary considers the quality and sufficiency of strategies for ensuring equal access and treatment for eligible project participants who are members of groups that have traditionally been underrepresented based on race, color, national origin, gender, age, or disability.

(3) In addition, the Secretary considers one or more of the following factors:

(i) The extent to which the services to be provided by the proposed project are appropriate to the needs of the intended recipients or beneficiaries of those services.

(ii) The extent to which entities that are to be served by the proposed technical assistance project demonstrate support for the project.

(iii) The extent to which the services to be provided by the proposed project reflect up-to-date knowledge from research and effective practice.

(iv) The likely impact of the services to be provided by the proposed project on the intended recipients of those services.

(v) The extent to which the training or professional development services to be provided by the proposed project are of sufficient quality, intensity, and duration to lead to improvements in practice among the recipients of those services.

(vi) The extent to which the training or professional development services to be provided by the proposed project are likely to alleviate the personnel shortages that have been identified or are the focus of the proposed project.

(vii) The likelihood that the services to be provided by the proposed project will lead to improvements in the achievement of students as measured against rigorous academic standards.

(viii) The likelihood that the services to be provided by the proposed project will lead to improvements in the skills necessary to gain employment or build capacity for independent living.

(ix) The extent to which the services to be provided by the proposed project involve the collaboration of appropriate partners for maximizing the effectiveness of project services.

(x) The extent to which the technical assistance services to be provided by the proposed project involve the use of efficient strategies, including the use of technology, as appropriate, and the leveraging of non-project resources.

(xi) The extent to which the services to be provided by the proposed project are focused on those with greatest needs.

(xii) The quality of plans for providing an opportunity for participation in the proposed project of students enrolled in private schools.

(e) *Quality of project personnel.*

(1) The Secretary considers the quality of the personnel who will carry out the proposed project.

(2) In determining the quality of project personnel, the Secretary considers the extent to which the applicant encourages applications for employment from persons who are members of groups that have traditionally been underrepresented based on race, color, national origin, gender, age, or disability.

(3) In addition, the Secretary considers one or more of the following factors:

(i) The qualifications, including relevant training and experience, of the project director or principal investigator.

(ii) The qualifications, including relevant training and experience, of key project personnel.

(iii) The qualifications, including relevant training and experience, of project consultants or subcontractors.

(f) *Adequacy of resources.*

(1) The Secretary considers the adequacy of resources for the proposed project.

(2) In determining the adequacy of resources for the proposed project, the Secretary considers one or more of the following factors:

(i) The adequacy of support, including facilities, equipment, supplies, and other resources, from the applicant organization or the lead applicant organization.

(ii) The relevance and demonstrated commitment of each partner in the proposed project to the implementation and success of the project.

(iii) The extent to which the budget is adequate to support the proposed project.

(iv) The extent to which the costs are reasonable in relation to the objectives, design, and potential significance of the proposed project.

(v) The extent to which the costs are reasonable in relation to the number of persons to be served and to the anticipated results and benefits.

(vi) The potential for continued support of the project after Federal funding ends, including, as appropriate, the demonstrated commitment of appropriate entities to such support.

(vii) The potential for the incorporation of project purposes, activities, or benefits into the ongoing program of the agency or organization at the end of Federal funding.

(g) *Quality of the management plan.*

(1) The Secretary considers the quality of the management plan for the proposed project.

(2) In determining the quality of the management plan for the proposed project, the Secretary considers one or more of the following factors:

(i) The adequacy of the management plan to achieve the objectives of the proposed project on time and within budget, including clearly defined responsibilities, timelines, and milestones for accomplishing project tasks.

(ii) The adequacy of procedures for ensuring feedback and continuous improvement in the operation of the proposed project.

(iii) The adequacy of mechanisms for ensuring high-quality products and services from the proposed project.

(iv) The extent to which the time commitments of the project director and principal investigator and other key project personnel are appropriate and adequate to meet the objectives of the proposed project.

(v) How the applicant will ensure that a diversity of perspectives are brought to bear in the operation of the proposed project, including those of parents, teachers, the business community, a variety of disciplinary and professional fields, recipients or beneficiaries of services, or others, as appropriate.

(h) *Quality of the project evaluation.*

(1) The Secretary considers the quality of the evaluation to be conducted of the proposed project.

(2) In determining the quality of the evaluation, the Secretary considers one or more of the following factors:

(i) The extent to which the methods of evaluation are thorough, feasible, and appropriate to the goals, objectives, and outcomes of the proposed project.

(ii) The extent to which the methods of evaluation are appropriate to the context within which the project operates.

(iii) The extent to which the methods of evaluation provide for examining the effectiveness of project implementation strategies.

(iv) The extent to which the methods of evaluation include the use of objective performance measures that are clearly related to the intended outcomes of the project and will produce quantitative and qualitative data to the extent possible.

(v) The extent to which the methods of evaluation will provide timely guidance for quality assurance.

(vi) The extent to which the methods of evaluation will provide performance feedback and permit periodic assessment of progress toward achieving intended outcomes.

(vii) The extent to which the evaluation will provide guidance about effective strategies suitable for replication or testing in other settings.

(viii) The extent to which the methods of evaluation will, if well-implemented, produce evidence about the project's effectiveness that would meet the What Works Clearinghouse Evidence Standards without reservations.

(ix) The extent to which the methods of evaluation will, if well-implemented, produce evidence about the project's effectiveness that would meet the What Works Clearinghouse Evidence Standards with reservations.

(x) The extent to which the methods of evaluation will, if well-implemented, produce evidence of promise (as defined in 34 CFR 77.1(c)).

(xi) The extent to which the methods of evaluation will provide valid and reliable performance data on relevant outcomes.

(xii) The extent to which the evaluation plan clearly articulates the key components, mediators, and outcomes of the grant-supported intervention, as well as a measurable threshold for acceptable implementation.

(i) *Strategy to scale.*

(1) The Secretary considers the applicant's strategy to scale the proposed project.

(2) In determining the applicant's capacity to scale the proposed project, the Secretary considers one or more of the following factors:

(i) The applicant's capacity (e.g., in terms of qualified personnel, financial resources, or management capacity) to bring the proposed project to scale on a national or regional level (as defined in 34 CFR 77.1(c)) working directly, or through partners, during the grant period.

(ii) The applicant's capacity (e.g., in terms of qualified personnel, financial resources, or management capacity) to further develop and bring to scale the proposed process, product, strategy, or practice, or to work with others to ensure that the proposed process, product, strategy, or practice can be further developed and brought to scale, based on the findings of the proposed project.

(iii) The feasibility of successful replication of the proposed project, if favorable results are obtained, in a variety of settings and with a variety of populations.

(iv) The mechanisms the applicant will use to broadly disseminate information on its project so as to support further development or replication.

(v) The extent to which the applicant demonstrates there is unmet demand for the process, product, strategy, or practice that will enable the applicant to reach the level of scale that is proposed in the application.

(vi) The extent to which the applicant identifies a specific strategy or strategies that address a particular barrier or barriers that prevented the applicant, in the past, from reaching the level of scale that is proposed in the application.

Sample Memorandum of Understanding

Partnership agreement between [college] and [school]
This partnership agreement reflects the overall commitment and the roles and responsibilities of [school] and [college] in planning, implementation, and evaluation of [grant name]. This partnership will provide 60 students with opportunities and services to increase standardized test scores, remain in the program, enroll in college, and persist to the graduation/college enrollment. This partnership [agreement entails the following for five years starting [date grant funding begins], and ending [date grant funding ends].

[School] will provide:	[College] will provide:
Identification and recruitment of students; curriculum assistance; assign program students to a single guidance counselor; help to identify and recruit exemplary high school teachers to serve as project staff for Saturday and summer programs; computer classrooms at the high school for faculty who integrate technology; assistance with parent recruitment and connections for workshops on financial aid and postsecondary options; student transcripts for all program participants at the conclusion of each school year and assist in developing a student tracking database; information about student college applications, scholarships, and enrollment; and cosponsor professional development opportunities for teachers.	A 6-week summer and a 20-week Saturday program with academic study in liberal arts and sciences; appropriate facilities, state-of-the-art computer classrooms tied to e-mail and the Internet, and other space needed for the program; a project website to be used by faculty, teachers, and students with links to appropriate sites; faculty who will assist program staff to develop standards-based curricula using national standards and city and state frameworks; visits to career-based sites integrated with the curriculum; services, including programming via distance learning and videoconferencing through ITRC; early college admissions testing and support for students as well as opportunities for qualified students to enroll in college credit courses; e-mail accounts for participants; creation and maintenance of student database with focus on assessment and evaluation.
[School] [date]	[College] Grant name [date]

How to Be Successful at Writing Proposals

1. Check in with your Office of Research and Sponsored Programs before you begin the grant-writing process.

2. Provide a draft budget and the RFP to the ORSP early in the process.

3. Begin to work on an RFP for a recurring program before it is released (usually 45 days before the due date).

4. Submit the proposal on time or a day before.

5. Stay well within the budget and allowable expense guidelines.

6. Be certain to address the funding priorities.

7. Convince the peer reviewers that you are knowledgeable about the topic.

8. Provide convincing evidence that there is a strong need.

9. Show convincingly that your organization has the expertise/experience to successfully carry out the proposal.

10. Consider the peer reviewers who will read your proposal.

11. Be concise but informative.

12. Redundancy is good, but repeated information should be consistent.

13. Use key concepts as takeaway messages.

14. Avoid typos, misspellings, grammatical errors, and such, which imply inattention to detail.

15. Take the time to read about and take notes on the essential components of your proposal.

16. Avoid including extraneous information to save pages needed for central components.

17. Provide information and definitions and define terms consistently.

18. Make your proposal interesting to the peer reviewer.

19. Use appendices only for requested information.

20. Respond in full to all areas of the needs section.

21. Provide references for the data you include in charts/tables.

22. Make sure your objectives follow the SMART format.

23. Check to see if the percentages used in your objectives are unrealistic, either too low or too high.

24. Assure that activities you propose are proven and fit the needs/objectives.

25. Be certain that objectives are specific and measurable.

26. Assure that activities are related to the objectives and meet the stated needs.

27. Objectives should be clear, specific, measurable, and appropriate to the project.

28. The goals, objectives, activities, and evaluative measures used in all parts of the proposal must match.

29. The plan of action or procedures for the project should be specific and relate to the purpose of the project.

30. The budget must match the activities and personnel costs of the project.

31. Provide support to demonstrate clearly why the procedures and activities to be employed will attain the objectives and goals.

32. Provide evidence that the activities of the project are feasible.

33. Make sure the section on personnel—especially qualifications, roles, and responsibilities—is clear.

34. Include a management chart to show how the project will be organized.

35. Provide information on similar projects, activities, evaluations.

36. Provide evidence on why the activities chosen will lead to the achievement of your objectives.

37. Data, percentages, and other information contained in various tables and charts should match.

38. The proposal should include all needed information.

39. Follow formatting specifications.

40. Show that measures to be used for evaluation are valid/reliable.

41. Clearly explain for readers the problems you cite and the programs you will implement.

42. Show that the proposal can accomplish its goals/objectives.

43. Promise what can realistically be accomplished.

44. Use the checklist contained in the RFP to assure that all required elements are included in the submission.

45. Begin to upload your proposal at least a day before it is due.

46. Provide sufficient time to for the ORSP to review your application, budget, and other forms.

47. The presentation of the proposal and the general appearance should give evidence of care and attention to detail.

48. The proposal should be visually appealing, easy to read, judiciously use **bold,** CAPITALS, and <u>underlining</u>. and use charts, tables, figures and flowcharts.

49. Avoid making the proposal pages dense so that it is easy to read.

50. Have others read your proposal and apply the review criteria to it before submission. You will be surprised at what they find.

References

Alba, B. B. (2016). *Incorporating course-embedded peer tutors in an accelerated developmental writing program*. Doctoral dissertation, Texas State University.

Allen, D. (2014). Recent research in science teaching and learning. *CBE Life Science Education, 13*, 584–586.

An, B. P. (2013). The impact of dual enrollment on college degree attainment: Do low-SES students benefit? *Educational Evaluation and Policy Analysis, 35*, 57–75.

An, B. P., & Taylor, J. L. (2015). Are dual enrollment students college ready?: Evidence from the Wabash National Study of Liberal Arts Education. *Education Policy Analysis Archives*. Retrieved from *http://epaa.asu.edu/ojs/article/view/1781/1624*.

Berger, A., Garet, M., Hoshen, G., Knudson, J., & Turk-Bicakci, L. (2014). Early college, early success: Early college high school initiative impact study. Retrieved from *https://ies.ed.gov/ncee/wwc/Study/84227*.

Campbell, D. T., & Stanley, J. C. (1963). *Experimental and quasi-experimental designs for research*. Chicago: Rand-McNally.

Carrell, S., & Sacerdote, B. (2013). *Late interventions matter too: The case of college coaching New Hampshire* (NBER Working Paper 19031). Cambridge, MA: National Bureau of Economic Research.

Clouter, R. (n.d.). Difference between project and program. Retrieved from *www.independent-consulting-bootcamp.com*.

Code of Federal Regulations. (2018). Available at *www.govinfo.gov/content/pkg/CFR-2018-title-34-vol3/xml/CFR-2018-title34-vol3-sec646-22.xml*.

Cornell, L. E., Greene, W., Haich, R. O., Mangum, L. C., Garcia, G. R., Guymon, C. H., et al. (2017). Proceedings of the 4th Annual United States Army Institute of Surgical Research Summer Undergraduate Research Internship Program 2016. *Journal of Translational Medicine, 15*(2).

Dobke, L., & Crawley, W. (2013). Strategies for increasing the efficacy of collaborative grant writing groups in preparing federal proposals. *Society of Research Administrators International, 44*(1), 36–61.

Donaldson, P., McKinney, L., Lee, M., & Pino, D. (2016). First-year community college students' perceptions of and attitudes toward intrusive academic advising. *NACADA Journal, 36*(1), 30–42.

Eagan, M. K., Jr., Hurtado, S., Chang, M. J., Garcia, G. A., Herrera, F. A., & Garibay, J. C. (2013). Making a difference in science education: The impact of undergraduate research programs. *American Educational Research Journal, 50,* 683–713.

Edmunds, J., Unlu, F., Glennie, E., Bernstein, L., Fesler, L., Furey, J., et al. (2015). Smoothing the transition to postsecondary education: The impact of the early college model. *Journal of Research on Educational Effectiveness, 10*(2), 297–325.

Feng, X., Chen, P., Liu, Y., & Song, Q. (2016, September). *Using the mixed mode of flipped classroom and problem-based learning to promote college students' learning: An experimental study.* Paper presented at the 2016 International Conference on Educational Innovation through Technology (EITT), Taiwan.

Finley, A., & McNair, T. (2013). *Assessing high-impact learning for underserved students.* Washington, DC: American Association of Colleges and Universities.

Freeman, S., Eddy, S., McDonough, M., Smith, M., Okoroafor, N., Jordt, H., et al. (2014). Active learning increases performance in science, engineering and mathematics. *Proceedings of the National Academy of Science of the USA, 111*(23), 8319–8320.

Giani, M., Alexander, C., & Reyes, P. (2014). Exploring variation in the impact of dual-credit coursework on postsecondary outcomes: A quasi-experimental analysis of Texas students. *High School Journal, 97*(4), 200–218.

Graig, E. (2012). *Hiring an evaluation consultant.* Riverdale, NY: Usable Knowledge.

Grant, M. (2016). *STEM-focused technology-mediated advising reform: Plans for implementation by four colleges* (CCRC Research Brief No. 64). New York: Community College Research Center, Teachers College, Columbia University.

Green, R. (2014). The Delphi technique in educational research. *SAGE Open, 4*(2).

Hauser, L. A. (2015). Precalculus students' achievement when learning functions: Influences of opportunity to learn and technology from a University of Chicago school mathematics project study (Graduate Theses and Dissertations). Retrieved from *http://scholarcommons.usf.edu/etd/5497.*

Hoffman, A. J., & Wallach, J. (2005). Effects of mentoring on community college students in transition to university. *Community College Enterprise, 11*(1), 67–78.

Hung, H. T. (2017). Design-based research: Redesign of an English language course using a flipped classroom approach. *TESOL Quarterly, 51*(1), 180–192.

Karabulut-Ilgu, A., Jaramillo Cherrez, N., & Jahren, C. T. (2017) A systematic review of research on the flipped learning method in engineering education. *British Journal of Educational Technology, 49*(3), 398–411.

Kim, J. H., & Bragg, D. D. (2008). The impact of dual and articulated credit on college readiness and retention in four community colleges. *Career and Technical Education, 33*(2), 133–158.

Kobulnicky, H. A., & Dale, D. A. (2016). A community mentoring model for STEM undergraduate research experiences. *Journal of College Science Teaching, 45*(6), 17–23.

Kolenovic, Z., Linderman, D., & Karp, M. (2013). Improving student outcomes via comprehensive supports. *Community College Review, 41*(4), 271–291.

Kuh, G. D. (2008). *High-impact educational practices: What they are, who has access to them, and why they matter.* Washington, DC: American Association of Colleges and Universities.

Kuh, G. D., & O'Donnell, K. (2013). *Ensuring quality and taking high-impact practices to scale.* Washington, DC: American Association of Colleges and Universities.

Lazarowicz, T. A. (2015). *Understanding the transition experience of community college transfer students to a 4-year university: Incorporating Schlossberg's transition theory into higher education.* Unpublished doctoral dissertation, University of Nebraska—Lincoln.

Lehman College. (2010). *Mathematics achievement with teachers of high-need urban populations.* Submitted in repsponse to CDFA: 84.3365, Teacher Quality Partnership Grant Program. Bronx, NY: Author.

Lo, C. K., & Hew, K. F. (2017). A critical review of flipped classroom challenges in K–12 education: Possible solutions and recommendations for future research. *Research and Practice in Technology Enhanced Learning, 12*(1), 4–26.

Moore, C., & Shulock, N. (2014). *From community college to university: Expectations for California's new transfer degrees.* San Francisco: Public Policy Institute of California.

Moore, P. (2007). The grants glossary: An educator's guide to codes, terms and tools. Retrieved from *http://scholarcommons.usf.edu/etd/5497.*

Morris, B., & Cox, L. (2016). Merging the mazes: Joint admission as a transfer student pathway. *College and University, 91*(4), 75–82.

Ni Fhloinn, E., Fitzmaurice, O., Mac an Bhaird, C., & O'Sullivan, C. (2014) Student perception of the impact of mathematics support in higher education. *International Journal of Mathematical Education in Science and Technology, 45*(7), 953–967.

Ott, A. P. (2012). *Transfer credit evaluations at New York State colleges: Comparative case studies of process effectiveness.* Unpublished doctoral dissertation, Fordham University, New York.

Ott, A. P., & Cooper, B. (2014). Transfer credit evaluatdons: How they are produced, why it matters, and how to serve students better. *College and University, 89*(4), 14–25.

Palmieri, T. (2016). *Lehman College mentoring program: Student Support Services: Careers in Teaching with the Educational Talent Search Program.* Bronx, NY: Lehman College.

Pell Institute. (n.d.). Evaluation toolkit. Retrieved from *http://toolkit.pellinstitute.org/evaluation-guide/plan-budget/choose-an-evaluation-design.*

Reinheimer, D., & McKenzie, K. (2011). The impact of tutoring on the academic success of undeclared students. *Journal of College Reading and Learning, 41*(2), 22–36.

Robnett, R. D., Chemer, M., & Zurbriggen, E. (2015). Longitudinal associations among undergraduates' research experience, self-efficacy, and identity. *Journal of Research in Science Teaching, 52*(6), 847–867.

Rothstein, A. L. (1985). *Research design and statistics for physical education.* Englewood Cliffs, NJ: Prentice-Hall.

Russell, S. H., Hancock, M. P., & McCullough, J. (2007). Benefits of undergraduate research experiences. *Science, 316*(5824), 548–549.

Sammut-Bonnici, T., & Galea, D. (2015). SWOT analysis. In C. L. Cooper (Ed.), *Wiley encyclopedia of management* (Vol. 12). Hoboken, NJ: Wiley.

Schultheis, S. (2014). *Evaluating an academic support program for urban at-risk college students at a private urban college.* EdD dissertation, Ralph C. Wilson, Jr. School of Education, St. John Fisher College, Rochester, NY.

Schwebel, D. C., Walburn, N. C., Klyce, K., & Jerrolds, K. L. (2012). Efficacy of advising outreach on student retention, academic progress and achievement, and frequency of advising contacts: A longitudinal randomized trial. *NACADA Journal, 32*(2), 36–43.

Sinclair, M. F., Christenson, S. L., Evelo, D., & Hurley, C. (1998). Dropout prevention for youth with disabilities: Efficacy of a sustained school engagement procedure. *Exceptional Children, 65*, 7–21.

Sinclair, M. F., Christenson, S. L., & Thurlow, M. L. (2005). Promoting school completion of urban secondary youth with emotional or behavioral disabilities. *Exceptional Children, 71*(4), 465–482.

Singer, J., & Zimmerman, B. (2012). Evaluating a summer undergraduate research program: Measuring student outcomes and program impact. *Council on Undergraduate Research Quarterly, 32*(3), 40–47. Retrieved from *www.cur.org/download.aspx?id=2842.*

Stephens, N. M., Hamedani, M. G., & Destin, M. (2014). Closing the social-class achievement gap: A difference-education intervention improves first-generation students' academic performance and all students' college transition. *Psychological Science, 25*(4), 943–953.

Struhl, B., & Vargas, J. (2012). *Taking college courses in high school: A strategy guide for college readiness: The college outcomes of dual enrollment in Texas.* Washington, DC: Jobs for the Future.

Susskind, L., McKearnan, S., & Thomas-Larmer, J. (1999). A short guide to consensus building. In *The consensus building handbook: A comprehensive guide to reaching agreement* (pp. 1–55). Thousand Oaks, CA: SAGE. Retrieved March 15, 2018, from *http://web.mit.edu/publicdisputes/practice/shortguide.pdf.*

Tsui, L. (2007). Effective strategies to increase diversity in STEM fields: A review of the research literature. *Journal of Negro Education, 76*(4), 555–581.

U.S. Department of Education (2017). U.S. Department of Education Office of Postsecondary Education/Federal TRIO Programs Policies and Procedures for Prior Experience (PE) Assessments Ronald E. McNair Post-baccalaureate Achievement Program 2012–17 Grant Award Cycle. Available at *www2.ed.gov/programs/triomcnair/mcn-apr-appendix-pe.pdf.*

Walton, G. M., & Cohen, G. L. (2011). A brief social-belonging intervention improves academic and health outcomes of minority students. *Science, 331*(6023), 1447–1451.

Walton, G. M., Logel, C., Peach, J., Spencer, S., & Zanna, M. P. (2015). Two brief interventions to mitigate a "chilly" climate transform women's experience, relationships, and achievement in engineering. *Journal of Educational Psychology, 107*, 468–485.

Weisblat, G. (2006). *Get that grant: Your guide to planning successful K–12 grant proposals.* Palm Beach Gardens, FL: CRP Publications.

Wellman, J., & Brusi, R. (2013). *Investing in success: Cost-effective strategies to increase student success.* Washington, DC: American Association of Colleges and Universities.

White, K. J. (2012). *Hitting the ground running: The social transition of community college transfer students in an admissions partnership program.* Master's thesis, Iowa State University, Ames, IA.

Wilder, M. B. (2016). *A qualitative case study on intrusive academic advising.* Doctoral dissertation, Northcentral University, Scottsdale, AZ.

W. K. Kellogg Foundation. (2006). W. K. Kellogg Foundation logic model development guide. Retrieved from *www.wkkf.org/search/site?q=logic+model.*

WWC Intervention Report. (2017). Dual enrollment programs. Retrieved from *https://ies.ed.gov/ncee/wwc/InterventionReport/671.*

Young-Jones, A. D., Burt, T. D., Dixon, S., & Hawthorne, M. J. (2013). Academic advising: Does it really impact student success? *Quality Assurance In Education: An International Perspective, 21*(1), 7–19.

Index

About the Author

Anne L. Rothstein, EdD, is Professor in the Department of Early Childhood and Childhood Education at Lehman College of the City University of New York. During her more than 50 years at Lehman, she has served as Department Chair, Associate Dean of Professional Studies, and Associate Provost for Sponsored Program Research. Since 1985, Dr. Rothstein has written over 400 grant proposals and received more than 300 grant awards. She has also directed many grant-funded programs for K–12 students and teachers and for college students. Her current research interests focus on college access and readiness, the impact of college readiness program dosage on student success, high school graduation and college enrollment, and the role of college student support in increasing 4-year graduation rates.